A Fish in the Moonlight
Growing Up in the
Bone Marrow Unit

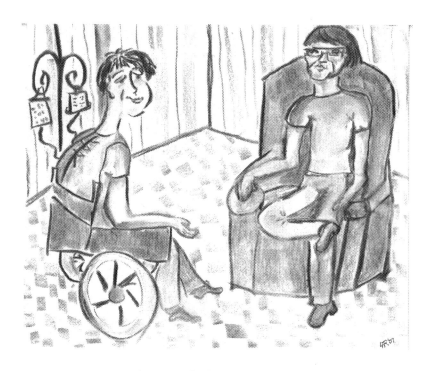

The Storyteller by Laura Richards

A Fish in the Moonlight
Growing Up in the
Bone Marrow Unit

Sidney Homan

PURDUE UNIVERSITY PRESS
West Lafayette, IN

Printed in the United States of America

ISBN: 978-1-55753-486-6

Libarary of Congress Cataloging-in-Publication Data

Homan, Sidney, 1938-
    A fish in the moonlight : growing up in the bone marrow unit / Sidney R.
Homan.
        p.   cm.
        ISBN 978-1-55753-486-6
1. Narrative therapy. 2. Storytelling—Psychological aspects.
3. Children—Hospital care—Psychological aspects.   I. Title.
RJ505.S75H66 2008
618.92'89165—dc22

2007042297

To my family—
Birdie, The Boot, and The Fictioner—
and to my dear friend, Dr. John Graham-Pole.

CONTENTS

Preface xi

Chapter 1 Tommy 1

The Baby Blue Bicycle 4
Mrs. Himmer and the Steamed Cabbage 7

Chapter 2 Did I Ever Tell You About? 13

Mama 14
Buying a Madman Muntz TV 19

Chapter 3 Christmas Eve 24

The Dixie Cup of Peanuts 26

Chapter 4 The Audience Grows 30

Leslie Doober and the Rotten Banana 31
Just One Piece of Candy 39

Chapter 5 Son of a Telephone Installer 47

My Father's Not Afraid of Bulls 48

Chapter 6 Uncle Marvin   55

Four in the Afternoon   56
Sand and Beans   63

Chapter 7 Brothers   73

My Dad's Pocketbook   74

Chapter 8 Being Different   79

The Black Sheep   80
They Never Asked Me   87
The Queen of the Mushrooms   98

Chapter 9 Something Good from Something Bad   107

Bruzzy the Bully   108

Chapter 10 Feeling Better   116

Going West   117
Staying with Aunt Grace   126

Chapter 11 Reality Returns   141

A Fish in the Moonlight   142
Put That Cigarette Out   157
I Envied Harry Lewis   163

Chapter 12 The Ever-Present   179

It's Bootiful   179

Chapter 13 Tommy's Girlfriend   192

The Smartest Girl in the Class   192

Chapter 14 Everything Changes   199

After Scotty   200

Chapter 15 Last Day on Charlie's Corner   207

The Casa Argenio   208

PREFACE

These are stories about growing up, *my* growing up, from elementary school days to the time I left home for college in 1956. They are as true as I can make them, given errors of memory, time's passage, and the simple human fact that sometimes, in unwitting defiance of the facts, we rewrite our own lives.

I've told them to my children at bedtime, indeed kept on telling them until, in their teenage years, they protested they were too old for bedtime stories. Then I started on the neighbors' children. Later, as an actor, I would use them as performance pieces in the theatre. And as Artist in Residence for our university hospital's Arts in Medicine Program I told them to children and their parents on the Bone Marrow Unit (and later to the teenagers housed on the Youth Psychiatric Ward). Here I relate my experience telling these stories to the patients in Charlie's Room, where artists on the Bone Marrow Unit perform.

Turning them into prose is something else. I do that here with the apology of Shakespeare's fool Touchstone in *As You*

Like It—they are "poor but mine own." They are growing up stories—an account of the formative years, of people, experiences, events, and places. An ordinary life, not important in itself, and yet perhaps for that very reason a life that may have some resonance for the reader. I am now in my sixty-ninth year. My children who first heard these stories have left home and are now fashioning their own lives, and these days their bedrooms, faithfully preserved, serve as offices for my wife and myself. I know that as I told the stories to the young patients on the Bone Marrow Unit they were using them as mirrors for their own lives—from the carefree days they knew before the onset of the disease, to that moment when the sad diagnosis was first handed down, then the hospitalization, the cancer treatment, to the present and somewhat unreal existence on the hospital's Bone Marrow Unit. My experience with them, performing for them, being with them, is ultimately more important than any of my own stories. I learned from my listeners, learned about them, and in the process, even at this relatively ripe "old" age, uncovered new things about myself. And for this I am grateful, "more than words can witness," as Shakespeare once said.

I hope my stories served a purpose, for this, after all, was my charge as Artist in Residence. For obvious reasons, I have changed some of the names and places mentioned both in the stories themselves and the recounting of my experience at the hospital. I will also confess there are times my memory has probably played tricks on me; if fictions seep in, they are inadvertent.

I've told both my own children and those precious children I met at the University of Florida's Shands Teaching Hospital, "If you wish, make these stories your own, and perhaps tell them at bedtime to your own children." With *A Fish in the Moonlight* I try to corral some new listeners—and readers.

CHAPTER I

Tommy

A button nose with a little boy attached, his head shaven, knees curled up, was waiting in a wheelchair in "Charlie's Corner," the lounge for families and their children confined to the hospital's Bone Marrow Unit—the saddest place in the hospital where I went once a week to read stories to the children. A diversion at best. Minutes before, I had turned down a request from the head nurse to help lure the children from their rooms.

"I'll just wait for them here, if you don't mind."

She brought a single child, this eight-year-old boy with the button nose. I had come armed with a Dr. Seuss book and two of my own children's favorites, The Hat *and* Red, Red, Red. *The boy stared at the floor, only on occasion taking in the efforts of the hospital staff to make Charlie's Corner look like a living room. There was a round table with a puzzle in the center, half started and then abandoned; a few books sitting unread on shelves at the far end; a window framed by curtains looking down on the emergency room entrance five floors below; and four shabby leather chairs that were seldom used since most of the patients came in wheelchairs. It was a laudable but sad effort to deny what the room really was, an appendage to a floor where children went to be cured, or to die. A dismal room, except for the huge circular rug with its faux Indian design, the clash of colors comic, even reassuring. No wonder the little boy stared at the rug.*

"Hello, my name's Mr. Homan . . . uh . . . Sidney . . . nice room." The boy's head sunk lower on his chest.

"What's your name?

A barely audible "Tommy."

"Tommy, that's a great name."

"No, it's not." He saw through my thin flattery, but at least he was now looking straight at me.

"So, what name would you like, I mean, if you could change your name?"

Silence.

A new tact. "You want me to read you a story?"

"No, my mother does that. She's at home. With Billy."

"Billy?"

"My brother." Then came the single sentence on which Tommy and I would build a friendship. "I hate Billy!"

"Oh, you really . . . I mean . . . your brother. After all—"

"I hate him. I mean it!"

"Why do you hate him?"

"You figure it out."

"Because you're here and he's at home."

Outside the sun was sinking, and since the staff had not turned on the lights, the room was now caught in that no-man's-land when natural and artificial light checkmate each other, the outline of the chairs blurred, the aborted puzzle indistinct from the pile of untouched pieces on the table, even the colorful rug muted. Tommy stared down at the floor as I played in my mind that last sentence, "Because you're here and he's at home."

I glanced at the three books on the floor to my right. Given this sullen audience of one, somehow Dr. Seuss seemed inadequate. I felt incredibly sad for this little fellow, here in a fraudulent living room while his brother probably sat playing a Game Boy in a real room near the mother who, having visited Tommy earlier that day, now entrusted him to a stranger, a story-reader who suddenly had no stories.

The little life he had revealed, his feelings for Billy, was now in danger of being snuffed out. And then I reached into what the poet Yeats calls "the foul rag and bone shop of the heart" and came up with, "You know, my brother John and I used to fight all the time."

"You did? You hated him . . . too?" He was amazed to find a comrade in brotherly hate. That "too" was the spark.

"Oh, yes, I hated him . . . well . . . some of the time."

Here was my cue.

"Did I ever tell you about the time we fought over a baby blue girl's bike?"

"No."

"Well, then, let me tell you a story I call **The Baby Blue Bicycle**. *"*

He moved ever so slightly forward in the wheelchair.

⚜

I remember that stupid little girl's baby blue bicycle. Why we fought over it I'll never know. A *girl's* bike, baby blue at that, a *girl's* bike with big knobby tires, its back fender missing, a rusty bell that didn't work, missing half its spokes and, worst of all, "Amy" written in bright pink on the chain guard. A *girl's* bike, and yet from the moment Mother bought it from a yard sale for us "to share" we fought over it. Our battles started in the morning and lasted until bedtime. We stopped for lunch and dinner, and for a few minutes later in the afternoon when we tried to share: I would get the bike for an hour, then John. But we even quarreled over who went first.

Each morning, right after breakfast, the fight began again. By noon we came to blows: I had braced myself against the side door of the garage with one hand around the seat and the other on the curved bar between the handlebars and the pedals. My brother straddled the front tire, his hand on the handlebars, trying to wrench the bike from me. We were at an impasse. For a second John seemed to give up—this was clever of him—and I took the chance to relax my grip and stretch my aching fingers. Then, with a sudden pull, followed by a savage cry of victory, he tore the bike from my hands, leaped on the seat, and pedaled down the driveway. I was after him!

Though John pushed the bike as fast as it would go, he only managed to stay an arm's length ahead of me. I ran as fast as I could yet couldn't quite catch up. Frustrated, I started to curse with all those words I had heard the older kids use. A volley of curses. Every once in a while, John would whip his head around and let loose a volley of his own. We shot those curse words back and forth like two angry cowboys in some western movie, guns blazing, chasing each other across the plains.

John made a sudden turn into the McMann's driveway. I was on his heels. Having used up the four streets bounding our neighborhood, we now raced through backyards, crashing into the shrubbery separating the houses. At one point John even threw the bike over a fence, jumped over it, and sped away. I took the same fence in one bound, lifting myself over its pickets with my hands tucked between my legs.

It was Saturday and our neighbors were out in their yards, gardening, emptying the trash, gossiping over fences, the morning peace now broken by the two Homan boys, John the pursued, Sid the pursuer—their prize, that baby blue *girl's* bicycle. Standing on the back porch, her hands on her hips, Mother cried to the neighbors she didn't give a "hoot" whether we killed each other or not, this was how we "paid [her] back" for all that she "had done for" us.

Suddenly it was over! John cut a corner too sharply and fell off the bike, which skidded into the street. I ran over, ready for the kill. Suddenly Jimmy Goff, a boy perpetually mad at life, drove up in his father's black 1949 Packard, a huge, black bulbous car that Jimmy, only thirteen, had no right driving. Seeing the bike in the street, Jimmy swerved toward the bike and crushed it flat. Only the bell—which didn't work anyway—was saved.

For the longest time, John and I stood there, glaring at each other. The first one to move, to blink an eye, to say something, would be a coward. Our faces were inches apart, and I could smell eggs from the morning's breakfast on his breath. We tried to rattle each other with cold stares. Could we hold these poses forever?

As the older brother, I finally gave in, telling John that if he was really that mad, why not go right ahead and punch me in the face. I had absolutely no idea why I had hit upon this idea; the words just seemed to come out of my mouth. Did I really expect John to take me up? Was I feeling guilty about having fought for two days over a *girl's* bike? I have no idea. All I know is John hit me so hard I fell to the sidewalk, barely able to hold back tears.

In a moment he was by my side, crying, begging me to forgive him. It was great! I enjoyed every second of his guilt. My strategy had worked like a charm. I put my arm around him and as we walked back to the house, I heard the neighborhood gossip, old Mrs. Schmidt from across the street, say to her brother the law professor, "Those Homan boys!"

Tommy sat thinking. "I liked it when you were chasing each other and when that kid ran over the bike. A girl's bike. A stinky old girl's bike. Now that was funny!"

The head nurse appeared, a sign I was to leave. Tommy saw her too.

"I'll tell you something else I hate," he said hoping for time. "I hate the food here at this hospital."

He meant the remark for me as well as the nurse. She smiled, having heard this complaint a thousand times. But I knew that his line was a code for me.

"Maybe next time I can tell you a story about the steamed cabbage I hated when I was your age."

"Tell it now!" he appealed to the nurse. His button nose pointed at me but his eyes fixed on her, "PLEASE!"

"Well, if Mr. Homan doesn't mind staying a little longer."

"He doesn't mind!" Tommy shot back.

"Just bring him to his room when you're finished."

Tommy waited for her to leave, and then maneuvered his wheelchair so that he was now sitting next to me. "Food you hated?" he asked. "What did you say it was?"

"Steamed cabbage."

"Ugh!" he cried out in mock pain. "I hate that too. Tell it!" Searching my face, he added "please?"

"Now this story is called **Mrs. Himmer and the Steamed Cabbage**. *"*

When I was nine and my brother John was seven, Mrs. Himmer invited us to dinner. Sometimes at school we used to play with Leonard Himmer, but we had never been to his house, especially not for dinner. Mrs. Himmer asked us to come on Friday night. We had heard from other kids that every Friday she served steamed cabbage. They had smelled it passing by on the sidewalk. John and I absolutely hated cabbage, steamed or any way, yet we did want to see what Leonard's house was like, how he lived. What was his family like—especially a family that ate steamed cabbage once a week? Also, the Himmers were famous in the neighborhood because they knew Frankie Carle, a bandleader who had once played in New York. Some people said that on their piano they had a signed picture of Frankie Carle. Of course, there remained the problem of the steamed cabbage.

We talked about it with Mother. She told us what to do: Be thankful for the dinner invitation, be sure to eat one helping of the cabbage, and then tell Mrs. Himmer how good it was. When it came to new things like this, we always did what Mother said.

At five minutes of six on Friday night, John and I set off. The Himmers were all waiting on their front porch: Leonard, his mom (who was very large and wore a dress that looked like it had little black beetles all over), and Mr. Himmer (who was very thin and long, and never spoke). Dinner was already waiting. We passed that picture of Frankie Carle as we made our way through the living room; it was signed "To my old friends, the Himmers—from Frankie and the Band."

The cabbage, in a big, deep bowl decorated with green and blue angels, waited for us in the center of the table. On the sly John pointed to the dish of french fries, and at the far end I saw a bowl of fresh green peas—one of our favorite vegetables. So I figured—and I knew John was figuring just the same—that even though the cabbage would be bad, there were still two things we liked.

First the fries, then the peas. I took big helpings of both. So far so good. My plan was to eat the cabbage first, get it over with, and then enjoy the fries and peas. John would probably do the same, because you know how little brothers are.

Mrs. Himmer stood up. "Now, boys, may I serve you some cabbage?"

"Yes, please."

She swooped over the bowl, tearing off the lid like a vulture. Suddenly the smell of cabbage hit us. The steam rolled down my face like an avalanche. With a big—and I mean *big*—serving spoon overflowing with the stuff, Mrs. Himmer approached my plate. I had carefully made room for the cabbage, turning my plate around so some empty space faced her. Plop! It almost touched the fries. She did the same to John. John frowned.

When Mrs. Himmer wasn't looking, I scooped up all the cabbage and shoved it into my mouth. It tasted horrible—slimy, stringy, like eyeballs. John did the same thing, and you should have seen the face he made. Still, the worst was over, and there they were, the fries and peas, waiting for us, like good friends. Since I had eaten the cabbage right away, not a drop of the cabbage juice had touched them. I was just about to put some peas on my spoon when I remember what mother had told us to do.

"Thank you for the cabbage, Mrs. Himmer. It was *so* good!" Not to be left out, John quickly added, "Yeah, it was so good I ate it first!" However, we didn't have a second to be pleased with ourselves, because in a flash, after a quick "Why, thank you, boys—I've never had anyone say something so sweet about my cabbage," Mrs. Himmer leaped to her feet, removed the lid, scooped up more cabbage, and plopped a second spoonful on my plate, and then one on John's before we could say a word. I looked at John, and John looked at the cabbage. From the other side of the table, Mr. Himmer, the one who never spoke, seemed to smile at us—slightly. What could we do? We ate the cabbage.

Now we were safe. Mrs. Himmer didn't put the lid back on the bowl, and as I choked the cabbage down in one swallow, I saw there was none left, just some juice at the bottom. Since the bowl was so large, I doubted she had any more cabbage hidden in the kitchen. The fries and peas were still there too, a little cold perhaps, but there. So, after I managed—*just* managed—to get the cabbage down, I figured I had nothing to lose. Besides, Mother would be proud of me. "Mrs. Himmer," I said so politely that John almost snickered, "that cabbage was so delicious that it's too bad you don't have any more, 'cause if you did I'd go right ahead and ask for a third helping."

John quickly added an uninspired "So would I!"

"Why, aren't you the politest boys," she said, motioning to Leonard who stared down at his plate. I think Mr. Himmer smiled a second time. "I do wish I had made more cabbage." She pouted, paused a moment, glanced up at the ceiling as if a solution were there, and then fixed her eyes on us, her face flushed with the sign of victory as she blurted out, "Now wait. I'll tell you what I can do." Once again she flew to the bowl and in a flash, before we could say a thing, poured half the cabbage juice on my fries and peas and the other half on John's! I couldn't believe this was happening. Leonard lifted up his head. Mr. Himmer stroked his chin with his hand. Mrs. Himmer stood behind us, beaming, like a hen waiting for her babies to hatch. "Go ahead, boys, try it. It's just scrumptious like that, poured over vegetables." We ate it. The fries soaked up that juice like a sponge; they were all squishy. The juice even clung to the peas. The fries tasted like cabbage; so did the peas.

My stomach turned. John looked green. Finally, dinner was over. We moved into the living room to hear Leonard play "Stardust," beside Frankie Carle's picture. At eight we thanked the Himmers for a "real nice" evening. All three followed us out to say good-bye. John and I walked down the steps, turned around, and then waved more good-byes. The big question was: Would we throw up before we got home, or afterwards? Then, just as we reached the other side of the street, we heard behind us a deep voice. "Glad you liked the cabbage, boys." It was Mr. Himmer.

~⚜~

"It's time for me to get you back to your room."
"I know," he said.

I wheeled Tommy in silence down the halls, past rooms where children, his cell mates, sat in beds, some watching television, others attended by nurses and physicians, a few with families who had decided to have dinner while visiting. The air was redolent with french fries and hamburgers. When I got to Tommy's room, a nurse relieved me. Tommy shook my hand, we said our good-byes, and as I turned to leave, he added his imitation of the otherwise silent Mr. Himmer.

"Glad you liked the cabbage, boy," he laughed.

CHAPTER 2

Did I Ever Tell You About?

Next Friday Tommy was waiting for me in Charlie's Corner. Once more, he was my sole audience, but this time his mood was different.

"Hi! I have two things to tell you!"

"Two things?"

"Yes, first, I don't hate my brother all the time."

"Good,"

"Now, number two—"

"Yes?"

"Did I ever tell you about the time—?" He became the storyteller, and gave me a wonderfully detailed, funny account of hospital food, about switching a side order of the hated collard greens for a custard dessert while his roommate Bennie was in the bathroom. And how Bennie ate the collard greens thinking they were the custard, the confusion aided by Tommy's fiction that Bennie was blind. The stories got more and more fantastic. Soon whole meals were being exchanged. A patient given five servings of split pea soup by mistake burst

into tears and went screaming down the hallway. A friend got three orders of the prized hoagie sandwich, and an enemy was stuck with a tray of stale saltines—Tommy's variations on "Mrs. Himmer and the Steamed Cabbage."

"I call that 'Good Food for Tommy.' Now it's your turn."

"Did I ever tell you the about Leslie Doober and the little duck?"

"No!" he cried, eyes wide, a fake look of anticipation on his face. "No, tell me!"

As I announced the title, **Mama***, Tommy sat back in his wheelchair, arms crossed, feet tucked underneath him, looking ever so much like an undersized Buddha.*

My entire universe was this small boy eager for a story. I thought of those Friday evenings in my boyhood, when my family gathered around the radio to hear our four favorite programs, the one evening of the week when we were all together and nothing else mattered.

We never took field trips at Cedar Road Elementary School. That was why everyone got so excited the day our fourth-grade teacher, Miss McClosky, announced we were going to the Philadelphia Zoo. "Tomorrow," she said, "we'll go out at noon and wait in the little area between the pond and the bus stop. The bus should arrive at 12:20."

When noon came, we raced to the little pond that made our school special. I mean, how many schools in the city have their own pond? We even had ducks; two weeks before one had given birth to five babies. So, there we all were, looking at the ducks and waiting for the bus.

Norma Roth, the kindest girl in the class, saw Leslie Doober standing all by himself. He was by himself because that's the way Leslie liked it. He thought he was better than the rest of us. Still, being kind, Norma walked up to him and said, "Aren't you glad we're going to the zoo?" In a very snobby way Leslie replied, "Yes, especially since mamá [he always referred to his mother as "mamá"] is going to drive me all by myself in our air-conditioned car." "That's nice," said Norma, struggling to be polite.

Leslie knew the rest of us had heard him, and so coming straight toward the group of boys where I was standing, he went on, "Yes, I'm going to the zoo, but instead of having to ride in a smelly old crowded school bus with the rest of you"—and with this, he waved his hand at us, as if he were some king speaking to his servants—"I get to ride by myself. Just me and mamá." Then for effect he added, "I bet I'll get there way ahead of the rest of you." Leslie always looked down his nose when he said "the rest of you," and he said it often.

Richard Fracas spoke first. "But we like the bus, Doober. We get to be together." "Yeah," Eddie Malnor chimed in, "and make noise and . . . and give the bus driver a hard time." Soon there were "Yeahs" of agreement all around.

"That may be fine for you," replied Leslie haughtily, "But I prefer to ride in mamá's air-conditioned car. Just me and mamá. I'm not like the rest of you."

As Leslie started to walk away, I saw Arthur Frank winking at me with a "let's get him" look. I knew Arthur had something good up his sleeve. Now, Arthur was an odd kid, as handsome as he was short. His coal-black eyes looked especially large next to his diminutive nose and mouth, and his voice was high-pitched, and always cracking. He moved with quick, decisive steps. Arthur chose to be the class clown. Usually, his jokes and pranks were without purpose, a strategy to draw attention to himself or to convert what people took as serious to something silly or gross. Once in a while, however, Arthur's humor took on a moral crusade. This was one of those moments.

"Say, Leslie," Arthur said, "While all the 'rest of us' [he said that phrase through his nose just the way Leslie did] are waiting for the bus, and you, of course, are waiting for your mamá—while we're all waiting, how about playing some games? You know, just to pass the time."

"Games?" said Leslie, not quite knowing what to make of it.

"Yeah, games."

"Oh, games, I *love* games." Then Leslie added, because he always added something, "I'm so *good* at games."

"I'm sure you are, Leslie," I joined in, "I know you're better than the rest of us." Only Leslie didn't catch my humor. Even Fingers Grittle took his fingers out of his mouth for a few seconds to smile secretly at Jimmy Neil and Spitty Grossman.

"Well, let's see," said Arthur as if he had just hit upon the perfect game, "Let's see . . . if you can jump up and down ten times on each foot with your eyes shut. Can you do that, Leslie?"

"Of course I can," replied Leslie, a little annoyed that Arthur would think, even for a second, that there was something he couldn't do. So, without hesitating, Leslie shut his eyes and jumped up and down.

"That was great, just great, Leslie," I said, motioning all the boys to join in with a chorus of "Great, just great."

"Now, lemme see . . . can you juggle two rocks in the air without letting them drop?"

"That's simple." Soon he was juggling two rocks just perfectly. Secretly laughing behind his back, the chorus sang out again, "Great, just great."

Arthur's turn. "Well, maybe these games are too easy for you, Leslie." He paused, as if he were thinking hard. "Hey, see those little baby ducks right on the edge of the pond? I dare you to pick one up." Leslie stared hard at him, as if Arthur were really so stupid to think that he, Leslie Doober, would be scared of a baby duck.

Leslie went down to the pond. We all followed, even the girls. He picked up a baby duck. "OK, that's not bad," said Arthur, "but now could you hold it tight to your chest?" Then I added, "And jiggle it up and down?" In a minute it would be 12:20; we could almost hear the bus coming.

"Sure, easy!" Leslie boasted as he pulled the baby duck next to his chest and started jiggling. When you shake a baby duck, do you know what happens? He gets scared. First he made a little sound like a pop gun going off, and then there it was—the baby duck went to the bathroom all over Leslie's shirt. *All* over.

At that moment both the bus and Mrs. Doober arrived. She saw her "precious Leslie"—that's what she used to call him— standing there covered with duck poop, and the rest of us laughing to beat the band. Mrs. Doober charged right up to him and screamed, "Leslie, how did this happen! How *did* this happen! That was a brand-new shirt!" What could Leslie say? What could anyone say? Something like "I'm an idiot for jiggling a baby duck on my chest until he pooped on me"?

As we boarded the bus, Arthur, making some excuse about one of the kids being late, asked the driver to hold up a minute. We all knew what he had in mind. Dragging Leslie by the ear, Mrs. Doober took him behind the car, out of sight. While we couldn't see what was happening, we could sure hear. We had heard it before, whenever Mrs. Doober got mad at Leslie. Margaret Bisher called it "the three sounds." First, you'd hear Leslie say, "No, mamá, no!" Next came the sound of his bottom being smacked. The third sound was Leslie giving out a little whimpering cry. Then it would start up all over again—"No, mamá, no" followed by the smack and finally the whimper. This day "the three sounds" were repeated ten times, and that was a record.

We looked back as the bus drove off for the zoo. Leslie and his mother sat in their air-conditioned car, all by themselves, without the "rest of us." Today, however, they weren't driving to the zoo. Oh, no, today mamá was taking her precious little boy straight home.

At the zoo a raccoon grabbed my camera when I got too close to the cage. Otherwise, I had a wonderful time. Everybody did. Leslie didn't.

"My brother came yesterday," Tommy volunteered.

"That's great."

"We got along OK. I told him about the baby blue bicycle, but I made the names me and him."

"Who got my brother's part?"

"He did. I was the one who tricked. You know, getting him to hit me and then making him cry. 'Begging for forgiveness'— that's what you said. Tell me another story?"

"What do you want it to be about?"

He was thrilled at the chance of picking the topic. A big grin led to, "A story about a time when you and your brother got along."

"I have just the story—"

He jumped in, "Wait, let me do it. Did I ever tell you about—"

I finished the sentence, "**Buying a Madman Muntz TV.**"

⟋⫘⟍

A few minutes before 7:30 every Friday night we would meet by the radio in the living room. John and I would each have one of those hourglass bottles of Coke. This had to last us for the evening; we used to compete to see who could drink the slowest, timing it so that just as the last radio show ended we would take the final sip.

From 7:30 to 8:00 we would listen to "The Lone Ranger." At 8:00 we listened to the detective show "The Fat Man," which always started with: "He goes into the drugstore. He steps on the scales. Weight—280 pounds. Fortune—DANGER!" During commercials and the station breaks, Dad would go into the kitchen to roast chestnuts, being careful to put a hole in their tops so the chestnuts wouldn't explode when they got red hot in the big iron frying pan. Coming back to the living room he'd slowly unfold a large white napkin and then throw hot chestnuts to John and me. We'd toss them back and forth, pretending we were jugglers, until the chestnuts were cool enough to break open and eat. At 9:00 we'd hear "This Is Your FBI" and at 9:30 "Sheriff Mark Chase," who flew around in a Piper Cub with his niece Penny chasing crooks. I loved those lazy evenings. Mom would darken the room so that we could make up the scenery in our minds. The world outside—school, the neighborhood, *everything*—vanished, and for those wonderful two hours, the bottle of Coke resting lightly on our lips, there we sat, facing the radio whose yellow dial glowed in the darkness as if it were a miniature fireplace. I liked to imagine that if you stepped outside our living room, you'd fall into deep space, a cold, dark vacuum stretching forever, held back tonight only by the walls of our house.

All this was to change. On May 1, 1950, Mother announced at breakfast that we were going to buy a television set.

"What kind?" John asked.

"A Muntz."

"No, not a Muntz," he whined. "They're the cheap kind. Why not a Philco or an RCA?"

We had read those ads in the local paper showing this ugly, wild-looking guy, Madman Muntz, pointing to a television set, promising to sell it "dirt cheap." Well, he told the truth because Muntz TVs were about half the price of the other brands. Still, I didn't want a Muntz for our first television set. Norma Roth had a Philco, and there wasn't any Mad Man Philco to embarrass her.

"A Muntz?" I protested, with John echoing me.

"It will be a Muntz," my mother said. That was that.

At 3:00 that afternoon the four of us entered the Muntz showroom, and were greeted on the spot by a salesman who had just one long eyebrow running right across his head. His hands were very moist, and he had a funny habit of looking down at his right heel every once in a while, as if he were checking to see that it was still attached.

My father broke a few seconds of awkward silence. "I'm Sid Homan, and this is my wife May Elaine. Boys, say hello to Mr.—" Dad hesitated, and then added, "I didn't catch your name."

Acting as if he hadn't heard the question, the salesman started to walk us over to the rows of television sets lining the back wall.

For some reason—I can't figure out just why—I stopped him and said, "My name's Sid too. I'm named after my dad. What's your name?"

Reluctantly, as if hiding a great secret, he said, "John."

My brother jumped right in. "I'm a John too. John Homan. And you . . . you're John?—" And there he left a space for the salesman to give us his last name.

When he finally told us his last name, we realized why he had taken so long. "John Crapp," he blurted out, then quickly added, as if this would help, "That's Crapp with a double 'p.'"

It didn't help. John and I could hardly contain ourselves. In fact, as soon as Mr. Crapp with a double "p" got into his pitch about Muntz TVs, John and I staggered to the other side of the store. It was all that we could do to keep from laughing and howling.

"Crapp! Imagine being stuck with a name like that?"

"And then he had to add "double 'p.' 'P'—get it?" I said to John. "Pee pee!"

"I get it . . . I get it." With that we started giggling so bad I thought our teeth would fall out. In a few minutes my mother began walking menacingly towards us.

"What's the matter with you two?"

"Nothing, Mother," we tried to say, our sides bursting.

"Stop whatever you're doing this instant and come with me. Your father and I have bought a television set, and I want you to stay close to us while we're signing a contract in the manager's office."

Just when we thought things were under control, everything went crazy again. When we entered the manager's office, there at the opposite end of the room was a large hairy man sitting behind a desk. Even though a floor fan blew directly on him, he was sweating badly. Facing us was a nameplate—"Fred Pew." Pew!

"Crapp and Pew," I whispered in John's ear as we staggered out of the office. We were hugging each other for support, laughing in each other's face, then moving away, coming back again, only to start all over, circling like two exhausted boxers, holding onto each other, waltzing in a stupor when they should have been punching. As we danced we improvised a song to "Crapp and Pew." Mother came out of the office—mad. She knew what was happening. With one stiff signal of her hand she ordered us outside. "Wait there, and don't come back into the store under any circumstance." She turned her back on us and marched away.

As John and I made our way to the door, a woman approached. Dad had taught us to let women enter first. So, trying to stifle our laughter, we held the door open.

"What polite young men!" she said.

Something crazed came over me. "Thank you, madam. I'm Sidney Homan and this is my brother John. And what's your name?"

"Betty Smell," she said as naturally as anything in the world.

"Glad to meet you, Mrs. Smell." We could barely get out the words.

Crapp. Pew. Smell. All in one afternoon.

The Muntz TV lasted just a little over three months. The picture tube blew a few days after our cat started using the back of the set for a hiding place, and—wouldn't you know it?—Madman Muntz only gave you a sixty-day guarantee. All that remained were those names—Crapp, Pew, and Smell. We went back to radio for a while. It wasn't that bad. But in the meantime just about everybody else in the neighborhood got a TV. I knew we should have saved up and bought a Philco, like Norma Roth's parents did.

CHAPTER 3

Christmas Eve

The day before Christmas when I got to Charlie's Corner the room was empty. I was sort of eager to get back home so I headed for the door. Just then the head nurse came in, with apologies that she couldn't get any of the children to come.

"Most are with their families. You understand?

"Of course."

"But Tommy was asking for you. He's in his room."

"He didn't want to come?

"He did, but he's not feeling well. We're trying a new procedure with him . . . changed his medicine. He's just not up to it. Now, if you want to—"

"I'll go see him."

"Last one down the hall, to the left."

"Thanks."

As I headed to Tommy's room she added, "Now don't worry if he doesn't talk. He'll know you're there. It's a pity his family doesn't visit more often."

"They do come sometimes, don't they?"

"Yes, but not that often. They both came when he was admitted, but since then I think it's been just his mother. When she does, it's not for long. Some can't handle the cancer. But he'll be glad to see you. Just don't expect too much from him. We're all hoping—"

Dwarfed by his bed, Tommy turned his head slightly toward me as I entered.

When he did rounds, Dr. John Graham-Pole, the wonderful physician in charge of the Bone Marrow Unit, sat on the children's beds. I sat down gently on Tommy's left side. He was so small there was plenty of room. I thought of that story by Franz Kafka, "The Country Doctor," where the physician actually climbs into the hospital bed to draw the disease from the patient into his own body.

"Tommy?"

No response. This was a silence quite unlike what I had known two weeks before when we first met. Tommy wanted to speak, I knew.

"You know, Christmas Eve is a time when all of us want to be with our families. This Christmas Eve reminds me of one I knew as a boy, years ago. A Christmas Eve when my father wasn't there." He looked ahead impassively.

I imagined Tommy was my son, and I was his father. I sat close beside him to tell my story. Later I realized that this

scene of father and son was the same formed with my father,
at the end of **The Dixie Cup of Peanuts**.

∽⚬∾

Christmas Eve! The dinner had been perfect. I was looking forward to sitting around the big, half-moon-shaped radio in the living room, a Coke in my hand, munching on those chestnuts that Dad would heat in Mother's big black frying pan, listening to a special concert by the Paul Whiteman Band. On this night I wanted the earth to disappear and my own world to be confined to that circle of yellow light from the radio dial. Mom would be knitting in the corner, the click, click, click of the needles so rhythmic that, John used to say, if you listened to more than ten clicks in a row you would be hypnotized. Dad would try his best to conceal the bottle of Schmidt's beer under his chair, for Mother insisted that it would corrupt John and me to see "Dad take a nip." Still, we would know from the rustle in the fringed cloth around the bottom of the chair whenever he had a drink.

Noses still tingling from that peculiar chemical smell of the city's water, John and I had just finished washing the dishes and were coming into the living room when Dad announced that he had some "business in town" and so couldn't join us this evening. "What?" I exploded, shocked, half in tears, "It's Christmas Eve! How can you go out tonight?"

"He has to. Leave it at that," John put in, followed by a threatening gesture from me.

Ignoring my brother, I begged Dad, "Why do you have to go out tonight—of all nights?"

"Sid, I've got some business in town and it's got to be done tonight."

A glare from Mother, who would never have been so polite if I had challenged her. Crossing to the closet, Dad put on his overcoat and the old felt hat that, no matter what the weather, he always wore going out. The moment Dad left, I screamed, "Here, John, take my Coke—I don't want it," and raced upstairs to my bedroom, slamming the door behind me.

I could hear the radio below. What good was Christmas Eve without my father? Why couldn't he have done whatever he had to do in town during the day, at work? How could he leave us now? This special Friday, the most wonderful Friday of all the Fridays in the year, was a disaster. All because of Dad.

At 10:30 I heard John come upstairs. A few minutes later Mother went into her bedroom. I couldn't sleep because Dad had let me down. Mother may have been the boss of the family, the one who made all the decisions, but, for me, Dad—Dad was the family's heart and soul. Without him, the evening, *any* evening, could not be the same. I lay there wide awake, staring into the darkness, seeing those pinpricks of lights cascading from the ceiling, little meteor-like particles that our science teacher told us were aftereffects on the back of the retina.

An hour later the front door opened. It was Dad. As I heard him coming up the stairs, I buried my head in my pillow. I hated him. I didn't want to see him. He went into John's room, to check on him as he always did. He would be coming into my room next. I lay still, pretending to be asleep. Dad came toward me in the darkness, then pulled the covers up to my neck, carefully folding the sheet back over them—as always. Then, just before he left, he placed something on my bed stand.

I waited until he was in his own bedroom before I turned on the light. There, on the bed stand, was a Dixie cup filled with peanuts, the sort of snack you get from a vending machine. I would have none of it. Dad's stupid way of apologizing for the evening. I couldn't accept any apologies—not tonight. It was hours before I fell asleep.

The next morning John burst into my room. "Come on, Sid! It's Christmas! Presents!" I mumbled something about not wanting any presents, but John grabbed the sheets and tore them off the bed.

"Let me alone!"

"Come on, Sid. You're gonna make a damn fool of yourself."

"What do you mean?"

"You'll see. Come on."

He dragged me downstairs. There, by the tree, stood Mother and Dad. I couldn't look at him, not even when he said, "Merry Christmas, Sid."

When I finally did look up, under the tree was the Deluxe Gilbert Chemistry Set that I had always wanted.

"You idiot, Sid. Do you know why Dad went into town last night? The reason he couldn't tell you why he had to go?" John was getting a lot of pleasure in telling me. "The stores were all out of that chemistry set. Dad had gone around the city trying to find one for you. Just before dinner he got a call from a friend at Gimble's. They'd found one more and were holding it for him. That's why he went downtown last night. You stupid idiot!"

I *was* an idiot for imagining that my father, the most gentle man in the world, could have done anything unkind. For thinking he had abandoned us on Christmas Eve. I ran to him, crying, throwing my arms around him, and he held me tight. We had a wonderful Christmas. The set had seventy-five different chemicals, five beakers, fifteen test tubes, a Bunsen burner, two microscopes, all sorts of plates and containers for mixing, and a thirty-page book of experiments.

That night, just before I fell asleep, Dad came into my room. As he always did, he tucked me in and then turned off the light by my bed. There was a new moon shining, and as I looked up at my dear father, his hair disheveled, his fingers, a musician's, long and thin, his body lank, and slightly stooped—looking as I myself would forty years later—I felt a love for him deeper than I had ever felt before. Without saying a word, I nudged the Dixie cup of uneaten peanuts across the bed stand, and Dad took one, before suggesting, wordlessly, that I take one in turn. He knelt beside my bed, and there, in the silence and the darkness, we shared that cup of salted peanuts. Neither spoke; what we felt was fathoms deep, beyond whatever words could sound.

To this day, every Christmas Eve I imagine that I can smell those salted peanuts. And see that dear man kneeling there beside my bed.

⚬—⫯—⚬

Tommy looked at me. I felt his hand touch mine. Seconds later he was asleep. I sat there for five more minutes, holding his hand, and then, extricating his little fingers from mine, got up and went to the door. I looked at him once more before leaving.

CHAPTER 4

The Audience Grows

On my next visit to Charlie's Corner Tommy had invited three friends. Teenagers, they were older than he; one, a fellow name Freddie, was very protective of Tommy. Freddie was loud and assertive, with a bloated face relieved by twinkling eyes. He treated me as an equal, and I found this both comic and a little unsettling. Grant was his opposite: quiet, reserved, respectful in the Southern tradition of sirs and ma'ams, an impossible lock of brown hair dividing his forehead, with a handsome face punctuated only by ears that, while small, seemed to stick straight out from his head. Grant glanced down at his feet every so often, as if to assure himself that they were firmly planted on the ground. James was a lanky teenager, built like a basketball player with longish arms, and yet incredibly graceful in his movements. His face had that pallor of almost every other young person on the Bone Marrow Unit. They were a mixture of body types and personalities.

Though half their age, Tommy brought them together; he had done so with stories, my stories, his versions of them. They knew all about "Buying a Madman Muntz TV" and, each in his own way, proceeded to tell me, as if I were hearing it for the first time, the gross implications of the names of the salesman, the store manager, and the old lady. "Crapp," "Pew," and "Smell" quickly led to a barrage of defecatory nouns and verbs, forbidden language, the teenagers' imagined passports to adulthood. At the crescendo, afraid of what the head nurse might say, I cried, "OK—that's enough!"

Freddie struck a bargain. "OK, but only if you give us a story," with a special emphasis on that "us" to remind me that now I was not just Tommy's storyteller.

Grant joined in, "How 'bout another Leslie Doober story?"

"I just happen to have one. It's called—"

"Wait—Tommy says you always start with 'Have you heard the story about?'"

"You're right," I said, but before I could say the magic words, Tommy, like an orchestra conductor, led the three new members of the audience with, "Have you ever heard the story of—" and then pointed to me for the title.

"Leslie Doober and the Rotten Banana."

Every time Leslie Doober did something bad and was about to be punished at school, his "mamá" always came to the rescue and took him home. When the rest of us did something bad, we sat for hours on the long bench outside Principal McFeeney's office. We didn't like Leslie. We called him a mother's boy. With a face like an owl's, though he didn't wear glasses, Leslie had this curious habit of staring at you with his eyeballs lowered, as if he had bifocals. We didn't like the way he looked. His fleshly body made it unclear just where an arm left off and a shoulder began, or when, precisely, one finger separated from a neighbor. Leslie didn't like us either. He thought that he was superior, until the fifth grade and the rotten banana.

The day before Christmas vacation, the clock said 2, and we were about to go to the closet and get out our "wraps"—those coats, sweaters, and anything else you put on over your regular clothes.

Our teacher, Miss Barndt, said, "Before we leave, boys and girls, would you all check your desks and make sure that you've removed everything. And I mean *everything*. Especially any food. We'll be gone for two weeks, and you know what happens to food when it sits and sits."

We liked Miss Barndt, we liked her a lot, and so thirty-nine old-fashioned desk lids promptly went up. Everybody's lid went up—except one, Leslie's. Everyone looked in his desk, everyone but Leslie. He was too good to do what the rest of us had to.

"Is everyone's desk all clean?" Miss Barndt asked. Thirty-nine heads nodded "yes." Leslie looked straight ahead. Miss Barndt didn't notice. She wished us a happy vacation. In an instant we were out the door.

Two weeks later when we returned, Miss Barndt started the class as she always did. "Is there anything you'd like to share?" Elizabeth Abbott showed us a porcelain doll she got as a Christmas present from her grandmother. Jimmy Neil said that his father came home on Christmas day, and this was big news because his parents weren't living together. Then, Arthur Frank, the guy who always made us laugh, put up his hand. "Yes, Arthur?" Straight off the bat Arthur announced, "Something stinks in this class . . . and I mean STINKS!" "Yeah, something stinks real bad, Miss Barndt." Joan Case, the girl who didn't mince words, went right to the point, "It smells like a rotten banana."

Miss Barndt remained calm. "Well, obviously someone forgot to take a banana out of his or her desk before we left for vacation." Notice that she said "his or her," because who knew whether it was a boy or a girl? "Well, let's just open up our desk tops—shall we?—and clear this up," she continued calmly. Thirty-nine tops went up. Miss Barndt thought out loud, "I wonder who left the banana in his or her desk." Notice again that she said "his or her." That's what we liked about Miss Barndt—she was always fair. "Well?" she repeated still calmly. Silence. "You know, there's nothing bad about leaving a banana in your desk. It's just a mistake. We all make mistakes, don't we, children?" Thirty-nine heads nodded "yes." This time Mrs. Barndt noticed one particular head, but for some reason pretended she didn't. "Who left the banana in his or her desk?" Silent heads turned toward Leslie's unopened desk. "Well?"

"Miss Barndt! Miss Barndt, Leslie hasn't opened his desk."

Not so calmly this time. "Mildred, I asked who left the banana in his desk and not who didn't open his desk." But we had all heard her the first time; she had said "*his* desk." She knew!

"Look, boys and girls, I'm not angry. Everyone makes mistakes. But I do want the person who left the banana peel to tell me. That's all. We need to find out so we can clean it up. Now, who left the banana peel in his [and then she made a point to add] *or* her desk?" Silence. Bruce Ramsey got out an "I know who it is" before Miss Barndt shushed him. Heads turned again toward Leslie.

"OK," she said forcefully, "I am angry now. Here's what we'll do. As I go down the rows and pass your desk, lift up the top and that way I'll find out. I *am* angry, very angry now. Not because someone left a banana in his desk," then came the refrain, "We all make mistakes. I'm angry that the person who did it won't admit it."

She started down the first row. We had forty kids in our class, four rows with ten kids in each. In row three, seat five, Leslie waited. Miss Barndt came down row one. In a way, it was beautiful—as one desk lid closed the next one opened. Lift and close, lift and close, like a giant bird flapping its wings, or a wave rising and falling as it heads toward shore. Up and down, lift and close. Closer and closer. We could all see Leslie look away; he knew he was going to get caught.

Now, whenever Leslie got nervous, he started twiddling his thumbs. Lots of us do that when we get nervous or bored, but Leslie did it a special way. He would twiddle one thumb to the right—the way a clock's hand goes—and the other thumb to the left—the way a clock's hand doesn't go. Try it—it's impossible. Both of your thumbs will go the same direction, usually to the right. Leslie was different—believe me, he was *different.* One thumb to the right, the other to the left, so that they passed each other, like people coming down the sidewalk from opposite directions.

When Leslie got nervous he also mumbled to himself, "Mamá . . . mamá." Leslie's twiddling became faster, his mumbling louder: "Mamá . . . mamá . . . mamá." As Miss Barndt came up to his desk, those thumbs were whirling like reverse spinning wheels, and the "mamá"s rose louder, more frantic, almost like a chant, until finally Miss Barndt and Leslie were inches apart.

"Quick, Leslie, call your mamá!"

"Doober's gonna be in the sewer!"

"Little Leslie twirled his thumb. Little Leslie, your time has come!"

"Quiet, class! Leslie, open your desk," Miss Barndt said firmly.

"No, Miss Barndt, no!" he whined in between twiddling and mumbling.

"Look, Leslie, if you did leave the banana peel there—"

"Mamá, mamá."

"We all make mistakes. Leslie, *open* your desk!" Miss Barndt's voice was no longer calm. Teachers in other classrooms, janitors in the halls, even Principal McFeeney in her office—everyone must have heard it. Leslie squeaked, "No . . . no," like a little spoiled brat. I bet he would open that desk only if his darling mamá told him. Now Miss Brandt was angry, real angry. "Leslie, open your desk this instant!!!!!!" From Leslie came a pathetic little, "No, teacher."

"I'll open it for him," Mildred Bosshart volunteered. Miss Barndt looked at her and Mildred sat right back down. Turning back to Leslie, still frantically mumbling "Mamá . . . mamá," she bellowed, "I SAID OPEN THAT DESK NOW!!"

Slowly, very slowly, Leslie raised the lid, and as he did a horrible smell rolled out and up around the room. Thirty-nine hands covered thirty-nine noses. Jimmy and Johnny, the Eyerly twins, pretended to be choking to death; Joan looked like she was going to throw up. Right in the center of Leslie's desk sat the grossest, ugliest rotten banana we had ever seen. It was black with green spots; there were some blue spots too. Hair, like that on a dead man, grew out from the sides. Little bugs were scurrying all around it. And did it smell! It was the grossest thing we had ever seen.

"Shut the lid!" Miss Barndt snapped at Leslie. "Class, quiet!" For a few minutes she just sat behind her desk, toying with a pencil. No one dared make a sound. At last she spoke. "Class, I am angry at Leslie, not because he left a banana in his desk. We *all* make mistakes," she said, looking at each of us. "No, I'm mad at Leslie because he wouldn't tell me." There was a pause. Then, "Now, usually, the teacher is the one who gives out the punishment, but this time, since the smell bothers all of us, I'd like you to suggest the punishment." The class was speechless. She said, "You." *Us.*

"Well?"

We all thought and thought. This was something new. After what seemed forever, hands started to go up.

"Rub his face in it for three minutes."

"No, make it ten."

"Let's all take turns beating him up."

"What about kicking darling little Leslie out of school."

"No, he'd like that 'cause then he'd get to spend all his time with his mamá."

Finally, Roy Grittle put up his hand. This was unusual because Roy never put up his hand; even at recess he almost never spoke. See, Roy used to suck his forefingers in his mouth while simultaneously twirling the cowlick on the back of his head with the other hand. Roy never had a free hand yet here he was, both hands up. "Yes, Roy?" said Miss Brandt, just as surprised as we were. "I think . . . I think—" Roy was nervous, that's for sure. "I think we ought to put Leslie's desk outside, just outside the sliding glass door. And I think we ought to make him stay there, outside, until the smell goes away."

"Yeah, let's make him stay out there all year!" Archie Leroy shouted.

"No, make it five years. That thing really stinks."

"Leslie, Leslie, made a smell. Now mamá's little boy's going to—"

"That will be quite enough!" Turning to Roy, Miss Barndt said, "That's a good idea." We all quickly agreed.

During recess, the janitor came in and unscrewed Leslie's desk from the floor. When we came back, there it was, just outside the sliding glass doors. Miss Brandt kept the door open a few feet so that Leslie could hear his lessons. Still, he had to sit out there all morning and all afternoon. When mamá heard about it, she stormed into the principal's office, but Miss McFeeney stood by Miss Barndt and what we had decided. So Leslie stayed outside for a week—a *whole* week—until the smell was all gone. We used to sneak looks at him when Miss Brandt's back was turned, making faces and laughing. Arthur found a fake banana in a store and brought it to school on Tuesday, wearing it on a string about his neck. Miss Brandt made him take it off.

⁓⊶⁓

Seconds after I finished, Freddie, Tommy, and James began a chorus of "No, mamá!" followed by the sound of a whipping, and then anguished cries of "Waaa!" Grant joined in, and soon I made the quartet into a quintet. We would have continued but the head nurse burst through the door with a "There are other patients, you know!" Five guilty boys hung their heads, promising to behave, as she turned on her heel; we fell to our chairs laughing, exhausted, chagrined, meek as lambs. In other rooms a child was deciding whether he should take the bed by the window or by the door. In another a boy lay quietly dying, his doctor at the foot of the bed having used up all options, now resigned to the loss. A teenager, pushing before her the contraption holding the IV, made her way unsteadily down the hallway, peeking into strange doorways as she passed.

But here in Charlie's Corner all was well as Tommy, three teenage friends, and I wiped the last tears of laughter from our eyes.

"Tommy says you usually tell two stories."

"I do."

"So?"

I decided to up the stakes by weaving a few spots for their responses into the fabric of the story, **Just One Piece of Candy**.

We never said anything more than "hello" to the Goldhursts who lived across the street—"hello" if the old couple were outside when we walked to school, "hello" if we passed each other in the grocery store. "Goldhurst" sounded German. We were just kids and the Goldhursts were so old. We had nothing in common.

One day we saw the Goldhursts drive away. We went on playing.

A few minutes later, John said, "Hey, Sid, look. They left their front door open!"

He was right—the front door was wide open.

"What would you do?" I asked the boys. "Stay where you are or go across the street?"

Freddie's "No harm in just looking" met a unanimous "Go across the street!"

"Let's go and close it." With that underground railroad of wordless communication peculiar to brothers, John knew that I knew that he knew that this would be a chance to peek inside their house—while we were closing the door, of course. I mean, we were doing a good thing because what if a robber came by and found the door open? We wouldn't actually go inside the house; we'd just peek in while we were shutting the door. That's all. Haven't you always wanted to know how other people live? What their house looks like? Especially people like the Goldhursts, people you said hello to but didn't really know? People with odd names.

Like a flash, John and I were across the street—we didn't even check for traffic—and on their porch. As we peeked in, just as we were about to close the door, we made an amazing discovery. There, sitting on a round table in the middle of the living room, was the biggest box of candy we had ever seen. It was red, shaped like a heart, the kind you'd buy on Valentine's Day, but gigantic. We took a few steps toward that box, our mouths watering.

"Let's take a closer look," I suggested.

"You know we shouldn't," John replied.

∽✽∾

"Go or stay and take a bite?" I asked.

"Take the candy!" The marching orders were given.

∽✽∾

Flash—we were at the table. Together we lifted the lid. Inside were hundreds and hundreds of pieces of candy, in all sorts of fantastic shapes. A few were already missing. And the smell!—chocolate, almonds, jellies, caramels, fruits, and creams. That candy spoke to us, "Take me. Take me."

"We shouldn't."

"Why not?"

"It's wrong."

"They wouldn't miss just two."

"We shouldn't."

We did.

John picked a honey nugget and I had a coconut cream. The chocolate shell, rich and sweet, cracked as I bit down. Then the cream inside poured into my mouth. The most exquisite piece of candy in the world! Probably from one of those exclusive shops on Vine Street.

Two pieces became four. Four became six. I had just popped a caramel in my mouth, John following with a chocolate-covered Brazil nut, when we heard a car pull up in the driveway. "The Goldhursts!" we panicked, our eyes popping. We couldn't leave by the front. The back door—that was it! Through the dining room into the kitchen. No! It was locked from the inside! We could hear voices in the living room. A young woman. "You know what they're like when we come too early." Then a gruff man replying, "Who cares? Sooner we come, sooner we go." They both laughed in an unpleasant way.

We were trapped! "The stairs," John hissed, and we bounded up three at a time. "Which room?" I pulled John to the left just as we heard footsteps coming. Hiding under a big four-poster bed in the back bedroom, we heard the woman say, "No, that's their bedroom. Ours is on the right." The couple put down their suitcases. We couldn't make out what they were saying, but their voices sounded irritated. The man seemed annoyed with the woman. We had already figured out that she was the Goldhurst's daughter. He was her husband.

Would we ever be able to escape? When the couple came closer, we could see their feet as they walked about inspecting things. We held our breath.

"What are you doing?"

"Just taking a look. Come here."

The woman's tan high-heeled shoes moved slowly toward her husband's loafers, an expensive-looking brand with ridiculous gold tassels on the instep.

"Look at all these silver pieces. Must be a fortune here."

"You shouldn't have opened their bureau."

"I'm just taking a peek. Get a look at all this stuff."

We could tell the Goldhurst's daughter was getting interested.

"Are you thinking what I'm thinking?

"Just one piece. They'll never miss it. Everything's piled any which way. They'd never miss one piece—believe me."

"I don't know." From the sound of her voice, the way she said "I don't know," she knew.

"They're old. They're not going to live forever. Anyway, we get all this . . . the entire house when they die. Come on. Let's just take one piece."

We could hear something being lifted out of the cabinet, clinking against other pieces. Then a drawer opening and another piece coming out.

"Hey, one, not two."

"Be sure to put them in the side pouch of your suitcase." The man had no sooner said "OK" when all four of us heard a second car drive up.

The couple hurried downstairs to greet the Goldhursts at the front door. "I know we're early but . . ." and "so glad you've come to stay" and "only one night?" floated up the stairs. Then we heard them go toward the back of the house, into the kitchen. A few minutes later all four were talking in the backyard. I snuck out from under the bed and peered out the window. They were wandering about Mrs. Goldhurst's garden.

We flew down the stairs to the front door. A minute later we were across the street.

"She stole something from her own mother."

"We stole something, too."

"Candy's not the same thing as silver."

"And Mrs. Goldhurst's not our mother."

After a few minutes, as if the same thought had come to us, we agreed that "stealing is stealing." "We're no different from the daughter and her husband," John pronounced solemnly.

"Forget it."

We couldn't. As we talked, we said the same old things over and over. John did point out that, in a way, we had broken into their house, although we both quickly agreed that didn't make us worse than the daughter. Still, I reminded John that what they said when thinking about stealing the silver sounded a lot like what we had said just before we ate the candy. The more we tried to separate us from them, the stickier our two stories became.

A half-hour later the daughter and her husband came out carrying their suitcases. Mr. Goldhurst remained in the doorway as Mrs. Goldhurst took a few steps toward them. When she touched her daughter's arm, the daughter pulled away and hopped into the car. As the couple backed out, Mrs. Goldhurst started to cry. After they left, Mr. Goldhurst walked over to his wife, put his arm around her, and took her back into the house.

"What happened?"

"Looks like they had a fight."

"Mrs. Goldhurst didn't seem to want them to leave."

"It's really none of our business," I reminded John. "After all, we've never said more than hello."

"And today here we are breaking into their house, eating their candy, and being there when their daughter and her husband stole the silver."

For the rest of the afternoon, John and I tried to forget what happened. We couldn't. It was just before dinner that we decided what to do.

Here's how we figured it. We could say nothing and let the daughter and her husband get away with it. But look what they did. Stealing from your own mother? Robbing your parents? Besides, the Goldhursts should know. If they made up with the daughter, she and her husband would probably steal again. Yet if we told the Goldhursts, then we'd have to tell them how we knew what we knew. About going through their front door. About eating six pieces of candy. About hiding under the bed. About sneaking back out the front door. Would the Goldhursts be better off not knowing? Something was clearly wrong between them and the daughter. Would telling make it worse? Something bad had already happened. You don't bring suitcases to someone's house and then leave a half-hour later.

The boys divided into two groups. Tommy and Grant insisted we should tell the Goldhursts; Freddie and James said we should keep the truth to ourselves.

"If we keep all these secrets inside us, we'll burst!"

We went back to the Goldhurst's house. It was difficult telling them the truth, about the silver pieces *and* the candy. But we did. Mr. and Mrs. Goldhurst sat without moving, once in a while looking across at each other. With faces worn by the years, their creases and wrinkles somehow made them seem larger than life, like characters out of a book. They listened quietly as John confessed to stealing the candy, after which I told them about the silver—just as we had planned. Every so often they would glance at each other, speaking without words, obviously knowing each other so well, having loved each other for so long, that a nod or a sigh was all they needed. I noticed their hands especially. Mr. Goldhurst's were rough, a workman's, his wife's soft, the color of pearls. How young we must have seemed! There was a dignity about the Goldhursts; they now met life in a quiet, unhurried way.

"I bought that candy to share with my daughter and her husband. They were to spend the night with us. We haven't seen each other in a long time." She had revealed an intimate part of her life. Then Mr. Goldhurst breathed deeply, "Things don't always work out the way you want them to."

We felt sad for these two old people with the odd name who lived right across the street. We hadn't planned to become involved. We tried to imagine how they were feeling.

When Mother woke us the next morning for school, there was a surprise. As we walked downstairs she explained, "Last night, after you went to bed, Mrs. Goldhurst dropped over." Had Mrs. Goldhurst told Mother about what we did?

There on the kitchen table was that big, red, heart-shaped box of candy.

"She wanted you two to have it."

"Did she say anything else, Mother?"

"No, Sid, she just said that you and John could make good use of it. That's all."

Over the next few days, John and I did just that.

CHAPTER 5

Son of a Telephone Installer

That night I called my brother John, something I should have done more often. The sons of a telephone installer, we almost never called, except for birthdays or Thanksgiving. We had not quarreled. Rather, as kids, each was "adopted" by one of our parents. The older, the more artistic—and temperamental—I became "Mom's boy." Mother resented Father for not making more of himself in life, for being "only a telephone installer," as she used to say. My father, a decent, loving man, was content to be bossed around by my mother. Both came from a culture, a time, where divorce was unthinkable: One married for life, for better or for worse. John became skilled in the very things for which I had no aptitude: mechanics, telephones, making home repairs, anything and everything practical. We lived in the same house but grew up in two different families, each headed by a single parent married to the other. John and I circled each other as kids, at wonderful moments feeling very close, but most often isolated in those two worlds. Worlds pulled apart further when I moved out of the house, and further still once John was on his own. For years, we never talked. What was there to talk about?

I decided to call John. We soon settled into a series of reminiscences about the good times with our dad, the comic events, most often those moments when he embarrassed us or himself, or both. "Hey, Sid, what do you think was the most embarrassing thing Dad ever did?"

"The most embarrassing? Let's me see—"

"What about the time he got chased by the bull?"

"And tore his pants?"

Have you ever heard the story **My Father's Not Afraid of Bulls***? You haven't? Well, then, let me tell you about it.*

Until my father was eleven and moved with my grandmother to Philadelphia, he lived in the country, near a little town called Embryville on the Brandywine River, thirty miles to the west of the city. At least once every week, Dad would say, "You know, boys, I'm missing that good country air. Let's head out to Embryville this weekend!"

Every Saturday morning, Dad, Mother, John, and I would get into the black 1938 Dodge my parents bought to celebrate the year of my birth and head for that good country air.

Dad insisted on driving five miles under the speed limit so there was always a big line of cars behind us, honking, screaming "go faster." But the other motorists never seemed to bother Dad. As hostile drivers blared their horns, Dad would turn and remind us, "Boys, every turn of the wheel gets us closer and closer."

The main street in Embryville led up a steep hill on the town's north side. At the summit Dad recalled, "Forty years ago a boy named Jimmy Feckles died right here when his Ford blew a wheel and crashed into that farmer's stone wall." The accident scene duly and inevitably marked, Dad would draw in a large breath, throw the Dodge into low gear, and drive through a dark, wooded stretch that suddenly cleared, revealing a line of rolling hills. He always parked beneath a massive buttonwood tree by the side of what had now become a dirt road.

Once unpacked, we always followed the same routine. We strapped big tin cans to our belts and headed out to the meadow to pick blackberries so thick on the bushes they fell by themselves into the can. In a little while the plunk, plunk, plunk of their hitting the bottom gave way to a fragrant silence as the berries piled higher and higher. We worked close to each other. Father would hum one of his favorite songs from the big band era, and since my brother and I knew all the tunes we'd join in.

No one else was around for miles. Years ago some big Texas company had bought all the local farms so they could ship cattle to graze on the abandoned lands, fattening them before selling them to butchers in the city. "The fatter the cow, the more steaks he makes, and the more steaks, the more money *they* makes," my father would observe, always with an emphasis on the "they." For several hours we'd pick blackberries among the deserted houses and barns, the sun so warm in the fields that, if you latched onto a clear rhythm in your picking, you would lose your focus on the berries and doze off. Behind a copse of birch trees a noisy stream made its way to the Brandywine River. Unwittingly preparing themselves for slaughter, the cows grazed in lush grass, indifferent to us.

In his efforts to give up smoking, Dad would suck on a little clay pipe, "Dad's pacifier" as John and I mischievously called it, a pack of Camels still bulging in his shirt pocket. Sometimes we would catch him gazing toward Embryville, recalling his first eleven years there. Coming to America with a proper British accent, the inheritance from my grandmother whose first husband, a London barrister, had died just before the trip over, Dad told us of being beaten up by school kids who taunted him for talking like a sissy. I knew that, for Dad, Embryville, the Brandywine River, these very fields were the source of memories happy and sad, but all his own, a time before the move to the city, before marriage and children, even before his own mother remarried a man as blue-collar and rough as her first husband had been aristocratic and sensitive. As Dad bent over to pick the bush clean, I could see the scar on the back of his neck, the vestige of his being scalded with hot pudding when at age eight he climbed up to the window ledge to investigate the contents in the big iron pot his mother had set there to cool. I wondered how he felt now, his life so changed from those early days, picking berries in the very field where, he once told us, thirty-five years ago he had harvested vegetables for a farmer who as a cruel joke paid him one penny for eight hours work.

Mother remained grim-faced in her picking. Clinging to the vine, defending themselves with thorns, the berries, for her, were the enemy, and she was not above instructing John and me—and Dad, for that matter—on the proper and most efficient way to deal with them. In the city I was clearly "Mom's boy," while John was relegated to Dad, but in the country there was no such distinction. The berries we picked, *all* the berries, would become pies or be preserved in Mason jars that lined the five wooden shelves that Grandfather, in his only act of generosity, had built for Mother in our basement. John and I had to pick four full cans before we had lunch; occasionally, we would examine each other's work and make approving nods. When we were finished, we could do whatever we wanted.

Sometimes we'd play hide-and-seek in the empty barns. One farmhouse had a secret passage on the side of the first-floor fireplace, which opened to a staircase inside the wall and led to a bedroom on the upper floor. Sometimes we'd dam up the little creek flowing through the meadow. Once we found a tire and took turns rolling it down a steep hill. After we dug a hole halfway down the hill, one of us would huddle there while the other rolled the tire from the top. Bumping and bumping as it went, you could hear it coming and then see it fly into the air inches above your head, its big black circle blotting out the sun for a second, before it continued on its journey, at last plunging into the pool of water behind our dam. Best of all was fishing with Dad in the Brandywine. "It's the fishing, not the fish," Dad used to say, as he gave us a lesson in patience. Once Dad caught a large trout—the biggest I've ever seen. But when he saw that the hook had snagged the fin, he told us he had caught the fish "by foul." Right there, he threw that big fish back in the river. "It's not right to keep a fish by foul," he said.

That same day, just about an hour before we had to go, Dad spied a big patch of raspberries on the other side of a fenced-in field. Mostly we just got blackberries and so we were eager to pick them. As we were about to hop over the fence to cross the field, however, we noticed barbed wire on the top and beneath the bottom rail. When we looked up, we saw why: In the center of the field was a huge bull pawing the ground, snorting like a steam kettle and looking right at us. We were scared, even standing there safe on the other side of the fence.

"I guess the raspberries are out. Look at that thing!"

"Yeah, put one foot in that field and he'll kill you."

"Boys, there's nothing to be scared of. Nothing."

"What do you mean, Dad? *Look* at him!"

"Boys, that bull's just part of nature. Believe me. I grew up in the country. I'm a country boy. I know all about bulls."

Dad insisted all you had to do was walk straight across the field, calmly, and "show that bull who's boss." With a "let me show you," and despite all our protests, Dad climbed over the fence, careful not to catch himself on the barbed wire at the top. Slowly, deliberately, *calmly*, he started across the field. The bull watched him. The bull did not move.

I had always thought of Dad as a quiet man, not especially bold. Still, there was one time when the Dodge overheated right in the middle of a one-lane bridge across the Delaware. As the drivers stuck behind us honked and cursed, Dad sat quietly waiting for the engine to cool down. It always did, if you just waited; if you were patient, the car would start again as if nothing had happened. The drivers became angrier, louder. Suddenly Dad got out of the car, turned towards those honking horns, and, in a very stern voice we had never, ever heard before, yelled, "Quiet, all of you! Keep your damn pants on! The car will start when it's good and ready!" The honking stopped. Dad got back behind the wheel. My mother looked at my dad in a new way. I felt so proud of him at that moment. I knew my brother felt the same. In a few minutes Dad started the car. John tapped him on the shoulder; when he turned around, he joked, "As you say, Dad, each turn of the wheel gets us closer and closer."

This time, though, we weren't laughing, because the bull, its nostrils flaring, was now furiously pounding the ground. I called out, "Dad!" but Dad continued in a straight line towards those raspberries, slowly, deliberately, just the way he drove the Dodge. Just as slowly the bull began moving toward him, making a lazy right angle with Dad. "Dad! Dad! Dad, the bull's coming!"

Glancing to the right, towards us, but not seeing the bull on his left, Dad shouted back, "Nothing to worry about boys. I'm a country boy. I know all about bulls." Now the bull was charging at full speed. "Dad! Dad!" we cried out together. Turning around to see the bull coming at him, in an instant Dad was off, racing towards our side of the fence, but only a few steps ahead of the bull.

"Lift up the barbed wire!" I ordered John who, like a dummy, grabbed the wire on the top. "The bottom, you idiot! The bottom!" I screamed, half out of fear, half from knowing just how dumb my brother could be, especially in emergencies. Dad was now about ten feet from us; the bull, about twelve. "Dive, Dad! Dive!"

The bull came to a screeching halt in front of the fence as Dad dove underneath the wire. Its bloodshot eyes bulging, the bull glared at us. As Dad slid under the wire, the seat of his pants caught, and when we dragged him towards our side, a big slit tore from his belt all the way down to the cuffs. We could see his underwear.

When he caught his breath, Dad admitted, "I guess I don't know everything about bulls, do I boys?"

On the way home, Dad drove even slower than usual. Horns blared. Fists shook. Dad commented, "Boys, it's all a body can do to keep his eyes on the road ahead." Her head buried in the map, Mother didn't say a word.

Chapter 6

Uncle Marvin

That Friday my audience had grown by one; along with Tommy, Freddie, Grant, and James, there was an incredibly thin man, slightly stooped as if he were apologetic about his height, with an angular, bony head, a perpetual smile that threatened to devour the rest of his face. He looked in his forties. It was his slender build that was most arresting. He couldn't have weighed more than 120 pounds, all this on a frame that must have been six and a half feet.

Tommy introduced the stranger with, "Sid, this is my mom's brother, my Uncle Marvin. Uncle Marvin's staying with us for a week. Do you know why he's here?"

Before Marvin had a chance to speak, Tommy kept right on going. "He's come to visit me. ME!"

I recalled the nurse's comment about how seldom Tommy's family visited him, the father only on the day he was admitted, the mother staying for short periods at best. I figured Marvin was the stand-in for Tommy's father. I learned later that Tommy's mother had sent out a call to Marvin who lived in California.

A little embarrassed by Tommy's enthusiasm, Marvin held out a bony hand with long fingers. "Pleased to meet you," he said before adding, "I want to thank you for my sister and me for being so . . . so good to Tommy."

"I'm pleased to meet you, Marvin. Have a seat."

As Marvin pulled up a seat alongside Tommy's wheelchair, the boy nestled his head under the uncle's shoulder. Marvin draped that long, bony arm around his nephew. Tommy looked at peace with the world. The three other boys grinned ever so slightly in approval.

"Marvin, you're our special guest. What sort of story would you like today? How about you picking a topic?"

Marvin extended his hands slightly away from his body, as if helpless when it came to making such choices. But when Tommy, still nestled at his side, looked up at him, sure that his uncle would know what to say, Marvin spoke up, "How about . . . how about a story about visiting your relatives?"

"Perfect," I added. "Let me tell you a story called **Four in the Afternoon**.*"*

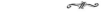

Uncle Willie's and Aunt Missy's farm in the country, west of Philadelphia, had a steep driveway and a wide front porch running halfway around the sides. Behind the house was Uncle Willie's shed. Years ago he used to park there, but now the shed was so full of junk that he had to leave the car outside. At the back of the farm was the "chicken hotel" with three floors, each floor having fifty pens on each side in a long row. One hundred chickens to a floor, three floors—300 chickens in all. Between the shed and the chicken hotel was the garden, and there Aunt Missy grew the biggest strawberries you ever saw. And the juiciest. Our aunt and uncle once lived in the city, just down the street from us, but Willie wanted to get away from the "bustle," and Missy had to have her own garden, not just a little plot but a real garden.

While the adults talked, John and I would go to the chicken hotel. The place smelled terrible, but, still, it was fun to walk among all those chickens. We pretended they were prisoners serving life sentences, waiting for a chance to break out, ready to grab us as we walked by to take us hostage. Putting our hand near the cage, we'd dare each other to leave it on the wire to the very last minute until the gullible chicken, running over to attack, would peck the wire instead. Frustrated at having missed your hand, the poor bird would stalk off to the other side of the cage and cluck.

Next we'd go to the shed. Aunt Missy was always afraid we'd get hurt with all the junk there, but Uncle Willie would simply say, "Missy, my boys will be boys." Uncle Willie, who didn't have any children of his own, liked to call us "my boys." Aunt Missy would smile at him in a funny way. He'd hug her, and then say to us, "Check out that wireless radio I got back in the '20s, boys," or, "Boys, I've got a hubcap from a 1927 Studebaker somewhere there on the top shelf on the left." We'd run off to find his treasures. The shed had no floor, just the earth, and it smelled of oil and rusty iron and leather. Though we'd been in the shed a hundred times there was always something new. Anything we wanted we could keep. Uncle Willie would always say, "I had my time with it, boys; now it's yours."

Before going in for dinner, we'd stop by the strawberry field for what John used to call our "early dessert." We'd eat ten, maybe twelve of those big strawberries. By the time we finished, the sun had started to sink, and Aunt Missy's dinner bell would ring.

Those were the most wonderful dinners you could ever imagine. First of all, there would be a big pitcher of iced tea in the center of the table. Then enormous helpings of "new" potatoes and green beans straight from Uncle Willie's field. Usually we ate country-fried steak, and rolls that Aunt Missy baked herself and which she told us came from a recipe used at the Parker House Hotel in Boston. After the dishes were cleared and washed—Aunt Missy always liked the dishes cleaned right away before "they had a chance to get familiar with the sink"—she'd serve strawberry pie with whipped cream. My mom always used to compliment her by saying "Now you can't get *that* in the city."

After dinner, we'd retire to the front porch where there was a rocker for everybody. Though we were just teenagers, John and I liked pretending to be "old fogies" rocking away with the four real-life old fogies. Dad would reminisce about his days playing with the big bands; Uncle Willie would match him with tales about the army, or running a grocery store in the city in the "good old days." Mom, who wrote a gossip column for our neighborhood paper *The Breeze*, gave the latest news of who was doing what and who was visiting whom. Aunt Missy was mostly silent, but she would laugh and nod her head in agreement, making a little humming sound in her throat.

About a half-hour before we had to leave for home, John and I would be asked if we didn't want to take a last stroll around the farm while the adults talked about "grown-up things." I remember walking with John behind the house, the hotel standing there dark and silent, the quiet broken occasionally by a chicken's throaty call, or the shed, its treasures locked inside for the night, waiting for the day to return. John imagined that under the stars the strawberries we had eaten were replenished by creatures of the night so that the next day the field would look as if we had never been there.

One night, instead of going out back, we snuck around to the side of the house to eavesdrop on the adults. We heard Aunt Missy crying quietly, saying something to my mother about wishing she and Uncle Willie had been able to have children. Then I saw my mother put her arms around Aunt Missy and kiss her on the forehead. After a long silence Dad observed, "But, Willie and Missy, you know you'll always have the boys." Then he added, "They think of you two the same way they think of May Elaine and me." After a second silence, Uncle Willie added, "Yes, Sid, that's a comfort."

We never called Uncle Willie and Aunt Missy before we came. We just came. Besides, we couldn't—they didn't have a phone. They could surely afford one, but Uncle Willie insisted that he didn't need the bother of a phone. "Besides," he added,

"I like to see people in person, and not as some scratchy voice on the other end." Aunt Missy would add, "Without a head." They'd laugh because, you see, my father installed phones for the Bell Telephone Company. However, being a country boy himself, he understood.

One Sunday in late September we drove out to the farm as usual, but Uncle Willie and Aunt Missy weren't there. And their car wasn't parked outside the shed. They were always there; they never left the farm. We looked all around, yet clearly they were gone. "Probably just out on an errand," my mother said. "Probably," my dad agreed. Then he added, "Look, boys, I know they'll be back in a little while, so why don't you go out and play while Mom and I relax on the porch."

In an instant, John and I were off to the chicken hotel. Though we had a great time running up and down the three floors, among the prisoners, still something felt different. John tried to assure me, "It's just because usually when we do this, Mother and Aunt Missy are in the kitchen getting dinner ready, and Dad and Uncle Willie are on the porch smoking and talking." Next, we went to the shed, and found some new things, as we always did. But once again, this time it wasn't quite the same. We missed Aunt Missy worrying about our getting hurt and Uncle Willie assuring her that "my boys will be boys."

The strawberries, however, tasted just as good as ever. John and I lay back and looked up at the sky, letting gravity do its job sliding that sweet juice down our throats. Above us the clouds swirled and swirled, like fat fingers pondering the world that stretched below them. John and I didn't speak; we each had private thoughts.

Then we heard my father calling out "Boys! Boys!" We ran back to the house. My parents were standing beside the 1938 Dodge, and Mother said that we had better start back for the city. "Perhaps they've gone on a short vacation. Without a phone, we don't always keep up on their plans." My dad still looked puzzled, as if he wanted to say, "But they're always here on Sundays. They've always been." All that he could do was repeat what Mother had said, "We shouldn't wait any longer. We need to drive back."

As I was about to get into the back seat, my mother reached into the glove compartment and, pulling out a pad and pencil, said, "Here, Sid, why don't you leave a note on the back door telling them we were here."

I got back out and walked slowly to the door. Stooping down and resting the pad on one leg, I wrote:

Dear Uncle Willie and Aunt Missy, We came by to see you today, same time as we usually do. But you weren't here. We had a good time. John and I played in the chicken hotel and then the shed, and the strawberries were good. But it wasn't the same without you. See you next Sunday, OK?

Love, Sid junior

Then, just before I pinned the note on the door, I looked at my watch. It was four o'clock, and so at the top I put a "4 PM."

Two hours after we got back to the city, there was a call from my Aunt Grace. She lived in a small town about an hour from

Uncle Willie and Aunt Missy. My dad took the phone. When he was finished, he asked the three of us to come into the living room. He looked grim. In very simple words Dad told us that Uncle Willie and Aunt Missy had died. While traveling home that afternoon on the Pennsylvania Turnpike, they'd been hit head-on by another driver who had crossed the median and ran right into them. Uncle Willie and Aunt Missy had died at about four in the afternoon. After hearing the news from the state police, Aunt Grace had gone to Embryville to make some preparations for the funeral. On her way back, she had stopped at their house and seen my note on the door.

That night John asked if he could sleep in my room. As we lay there in the dark we talked about Uncle Willie and Aunt Missy. About their not being able to have children. About the country-fried steak and new potatoes. About the strawberry field. And the chicken hotel. About the treasures in the shed. About being Uncle Willie's "boys." Then we tried to fall asleep, each pretending, for the sake of the other, that we had.

⌒╫⌒

No sooner had I finished then I regretted my choice, my telling a story that ended with death. The kids picked up on the issue right away.

"It's crazy. At the same time you were writing that note they were being killed."

"Did you ever get to sleep or did you just stay up all night worrying?"

I felt like an idiot, here where the patients knew an empty bed meant either someone had gone home or had died. I looked to Marvin to rescue me.

"I bet Mr. Homan has another story."

I grabbed the opportunity. Something light. The kids had now grown very solemn. I asked, "Did I ever tell you the story about **Sand and Beans***?"*

⁓❦⁓

My children call it "Dad's sand phobia." Before I get into bed and put my feet under the covers, I must wipe them three times—not just two, or one, but three. If I get out of bed and return, before I can get back in, I have to wipe my feet—three times. It doesn't make any difference whether I wear bedroom slippers, socks, or try to step lightly. I must always clean my feet if I get out of bed. If I forget to do so or if I purposely try not to clean my feet, I can't sleep but, instead, toss and turn in my bed, imagining grains of sand clinging to me. To this day, whether staying high in the mountains, at sea, even in a state that has no beaches, on Georgia clay, no matter where, I imagine sand lurks—on the floor, near my feet—waiting to be carried back into my bed.

It's all because of Wildwood-by-the-Sea on the Jersey coast. During our one-week vacation there we always stayed at the same place, the Poretta's cottage. It was run-down, with so many cracks in the floor that the sand came pouring in. Overwhelmed by a large shed that was off-limits to us, the yard was absolutely bare, without a single tree, not even a bush. But there was plenty of sand. Now my mother had this notion that since you paid to go on vacation, you were paying to have fun. In Wildwood fun meant waves and sand, and so each day we would leave for the beach at sunrise and stay until sunset. Twelve hours a day, seven days, surrounded by sand. Back at the Poretta's cottage, more sand. Sand everywhere. Under toenails, in food, in my mouth, on my skin, and always in *my* bed.

We never saw the Porettas. For all I knew, they could have been figments of my mother's imagination. Still, we always stayed at their cottage. It was the custom in Wildwood to give such rental places cute names, a way of attracting customers, making the place seem more homey. So, up and down the street you'd pass cottages with signs on the door or stuck in the lawn announcing "The Welcome Inn" or "Betty's-By-The-Beach" or "Wilma's Bellweather." As far as I was concerned, the Porettas should have named their place "Sand Trap."

To make it through those long days on the beach, John and I played in the surf, challenging each other by leaping over waves. We took long, long walks along the shore, and, as the years passed, began to notice girls in bathing suits, trying, but failing, to be casual while staring. We constructed sand castles where the waves hit the shore, desperately building bigger and bigger walls to ward off the sea. I buried John in sand; he never, of course, buried me. We made miniature golf courses where we played with croquet balls and mallets. If the wind was blowing that day from the ocean, everything was fine, but if it came from the land, then you got bit by those big Jersey mosquitoes. At noon, Mom took lunch out of the picnic basket and that helped break up the long day. However, she always served sardine sandwiches on Tuesdays and Thursdays. "Nourishing" was Mother's only response when we were so bold as to question her menu.

The days at the beach were long, too long, with few surprises. One diversion was exploring underneath the boardwalk that ran for almost two miles, separating the beach from the stores and amusements. You could occasionally find money that dropped down from people's pockets or had slipped through their fingers. One day while we were searching we heard two guys start to argue right above our heads. We couldn't see them, except for an occasional glimpse of a shoe between the cracks in the wood. But we could sure hear them. They were screaming; soon those screams gave way to a real knock-down, drag-out fistfight. One of the guys fell and the other jumped on top of him. Rolling about the boardwalk, right over our heads, they were punching away at each other.

"Look, Sid!" John shouted. He had just seen two coins slip through the cracks and fall to the sand. In a flash we had dug them out. Two more coins; then another, and at length a whole handful. In a few minutes John and I had collected six dollars, and considering this was 1951 and that money was worth more, you'd have to multiply by ten to get some idea of why we were so excited.

All at once the coins stopped falling. Above us, the guys were apologizing to each other. They were brothers, like us. A few seconds later, one of them cried, "Where's my money?" "Mine's gone too. Must have dropped out while we were fighting."

"Let's get out of here," I said.

"Which way?'

"Back to where Mother and Dad are!"

We were off. Without stopping, I turned around and saw the two guys coming down the steps leading from the boardwalk to the beach. One of them must have looked in our direction. "Hey, those two kids, they've got our money!" We knew they would be after us any second.

John and I saw our parents ahead in the water. Around them were several families with kids. We knew what to do! Racing towards the crowd, soon we were splashing around in the surf as if nothing had happened, as if we had been there all the time.

"What'll I do with the money?" John asked. "My bathing suit doesn't have a pocket!"

"Put it in your mouth." That's all I could think of. So, as the two guys came racing up, there John and I were innocently playing, trying to blend in with the families, the six dollars in our mouths, our cheeks puffed out. The brothers wandered around for a while, afraid to ask parents if they could check and see if their kids had the money, but hoping for some clue, like a bulging bathing-suit pocket. After a while, they went away, mad no doubt. That day at the beach didn't seem quite as long as usual.

The nights, now the nights were a different story entirely. As soon as the supper dishes were cleaned and put away, Mother would give John and me a dollar each for the boardwalk. It was a long walk from the Porettas but at least we were on our own, with that dollar sitting happily in our pockets. Along the beach, the boardwalk stretched as wide as an eight-lane highway. On the east side lay the dark ocean which you couldn't see, although once in a while, between the noise of the people and the rides, you could hear waves breaking. On the other side were stores, amusement rides, salt water taffy shops, showplaces, concession stands, and lights, lights everywhere. Nature, dark and expectant on the one side, and on the other neon lights challenging the night.

The Nickel-o-rama was always the first place we went. For five cents you could try to win a prize at skee-ball, get your fortune told by a mechanical lady in a glass case, play golf on a four-hole course no bigger than a small table, or work the pinball machines (which tilted at the slightest touch). You could test your strength on the hand-grip, or—if you were careful that no one, especially a brother, was looking over your shoulder—rate your "love life" by pushing buttons to answer questions from a machine. John and I usually spent about twenty-five cents in the Nickel-o-rama before getting a mile-long hot dog, with the sauerkraut piled high, and a Coke in a glass bottle for twenty-five cents. So far, fifty cents, and the evening was only a third over.

The last fifty cents went for rides. The rickety wooden roller coaster, or the "Ocean Drop," the only ride on the beach side, where you stood with your back against the inside wall of a barrel, facing its center. Once that barrel started rotating fast enough, the bottom dropped out. Fifty feet below you was the ocean, but you didn't fall because of the force pinning you against the wall. The "Spook House" had collapsible stairs and a dark room where little hands rubbed against your ankles. In the "Bump-'d-Bump" we smashed into each other in automobiles powered by lawnmower engines.

Best of all was the "Hall of Mirrors," a maze in which the trick was to find the one "wall" in a particular room—and every room had three, four, five, or even more walls—that was not really solid, not glass, but an entrance to the next room. You'd think it would be easy to discover the entrance by feeling around, but somehow, when you were in the maze, glass reflecting off glass so that the air itself seemed to be a mirror, panic set in. The crowd surrounding the maze laughed as people bumped into walls and purposely confused them by calling out conflicting advice. For those impossibly lost, a midget, who knew the maze like the back of his hand, would come to the rescue, leading the embarrassed customer to the exit like some naughty child.

Mother and Dad seemed far away. I hoped those nights at the boardwalk would never end. I dreamed that outside the bright strip of lights, beyond the amusements, the everyday world, Wildwood, and especially the Poretta's cottage, had vanished.

At 10:30 we had to go back to "The Sand Trap." John and I always started in high spirits, reviewing the events of the evening, comparing the present night to its predecessors. As we neared the Poretta's cottage, though, my mood would change. I began worrying about the sand, about trying to fall asleep, knowing that no matter how carefully I showered, even washing my feet before bed, somewhere under the covers, perhaps carried to the bed under my fingernail, would be the single grain of sand, the pea that the princess could feel under twenty pillows, and that would keep me tossing and turning until fatigue set in, just before dawn, just before Mother's cheery "Rise and shine, boys," signaling yet another grainy day at the beach.

On the seventh day we would prepare for the trip back to the city, the *long* trip back given my father's insistence on traveling five miles per hour under the speed limit. We always took the same route, cutting a diagonal across the state, then making our way through the city, our home just a few miles away, being slowed down by stops at almost every block since the traffic lights on Broad Street never seemed to be synchronized.

Only once did we take a different route. It was Dad's idea, and since he loved the predictable and hated change, we were shocked when he suggested that we travel north, along the Delaware, before crossing over to Philly.

After an hour on the "new" route it became clear that we were the sole car on a narrow, two-lane road making its way through mile after mile of scruffy pine. A half-hour later we were hungry, but there was no restaurant in sight, indeed, no sign of any life at all. From the back seat I began complaining; from the front, Mother reminded Dad, as if he needed reminding, of the consequences of his radical decision. Of course, even though the road was deserted, Dad kept to his principle of five miles under the speed limit. It was maddening.

I feared we would spend eternity on this back road, starving to death, our bones sinking into the dust along the road, the sand in Poretta's cottage greedily anticipating its next victim. However, just when all seemed hopeless, a restaurant appeared. On all other occasions Dad was conservative to a fault with his 1938 Dodge; this time he threw on the brakes, and the car ground to an unaccustomed quick stop.

Small and unpretentious, the restaurant had a single room, eight tables, with no one in sight. The walls were bare; the tables were bare, except for one in the center of the room, set for four. For us! We sat and, in a few minutes, a family of three appeared, pleasant looking people and amazingly alike. The son, maybe eight or nine, introduced his mother and father, "the Sledges." For a few minutes, we made small talk—the loneliness of the road, the fun we had at the beach (or so Mother insisted).

"May we see a menu?" My mother got right down to business.

"Menu?" an astonished Mrs. Sledge replied.

Her husband apologized. "We don't have a menu." Then, more affirmatively, "Never had."

My father, the diplomat, the "peacemaker" as he liked to call himself, asked, "What *are* you serving tonight?" The question sounded old-fashioned.

As one, the three Sledges replied, "Beans."

"Beans," we four Homans said to ourselves, although some involuntary movement in the lips must have given away our surprise, even alarm, for Mrs. Sledge quickly added, "*Baked* beans," as if the adjective might rescue the occasion.

"Then beans it will be," I replied, knowing that my family, once they had committed themselves to the table, would never back down.

"For four," John added, being at once helpful and obvious.

Minutes later the beans arrived. Bean soup, bean casserole (whose only ingredient seemed to be beans), the promised main course of baked beans, and, for desert, bean custard made from beans laced with sugar. *Beans.*

For the duration of the meal the Sledges sat at a nearby table, chatting with us. A complete family history unfurled. They liked the solitude of the place, were essentially self-supporting. Attracting only lost souls and families, like our own, who had decided to take the back ways, the restaurant brought the most modest income, just enough cash to buy what the Sledges themselves could not grow or make or repair.

Despite the beans—for caught up in the conversation we forgot the monotony of the meal—we spent a pleasant hour. A meeting between two families, doubtless the *only* meeting the two families would ever have. A few years later, Miss Chew, my ninth-grade Latin teacher, would tell us that in those deserted, far-flung reaches of the Empire, when two Romans passed each other on the road, without slowing their pace they would say to each other, "Salve," followed by an "Atque vale." "Hello" and "Farewell." The Homans and the Sledges were such passers-by.

As we drove off, we were quiet until from the back seat John suggested, "Next year, Dad, let's take the regular way back." Then, to much laughter from John and me, with cold stares from my mother directed to us, and with Dad, as usual, smiling quietly to himself, the beans spoke.

❧

And the boys and Marvin spoke too—with their laughter at the thought of my prissy mother having to endure the long ride home—with only the beans talking.

Chapter 7

Brothers

Everything changes. Two weeks ago I had called my brother for the first time in years. The next week he called me, and I told John about Charlie's Corner, about the young people, about how I was using stories about me, about him, about our family, our own growing up. He was delighted to hear about their reaction to "My Father's Not Afraid of Bulls."

"I bet they laughed when his pants tore on the fence."

"Laugh? You should have heard them, John. And they laughed when I told them about how you lifted up the top of the barbed wire when I meant the bottom."

"I thought I was the one who told you to do that," he joked, and then added, "I can see Dad's underwear as if it were yesterday."

I could picture and even feel John over the phone, the way a phone conversation between two people who know each other well is very different from one with strangers. You're used to each other's rhythms, the expression that invariably accompanies this or that phrase. I knew what John was feeling. I

searched for a memory, a story where all four Homans were
present, one that John and I shared with both Mom and Dad.

"John, do you remember the time Dad called his wallet his
pocketbook?"

⚜

My Dad's Pocketbook

No sooner had we sat down then a waiter practically rushed up to the table, placing a board of freshly made bread in the center and small dishes of mint-flavored coleslaw at our places. One moment he introduced himself as Alfred, the next he was off to the kitchen—I suppose to bring menus. We were all hungry and before he reappeared the bread and the coleslaw were gone.

"My, we were hungry, weren't we?" he said in a fairly sarcastic way on returning. Mother glared at him. She had this notion that since waiters were only "servants" (as she called them) and were therefore not your "social equals" (again, her phrase), they should never, under any circumstances, engage in conversation with customers. Dad had no such notion but, instead, as if now obliged to reply, said in a wonderfully innocent way, "Best place to be hungry is a restaurant, ain't it?" On the spot, the snobby waiter was transformed. With a kindly "Now that's the truth," he swooped around the table handing us the menus. On Dad's attempt at familiarity, however, Mother glared again, and glared a third time when, looking at the menu, he whispered to her, "May Elaine, get a look at these prices."

Dad was right—the prices were out of this world.

"What should we do?"

"Well, Sidney, we sure can't stay," she replied, purposely mocking his name with the more formal "Sidney."

"But we've already eaten their bread and the coleslaw."

"Their? *Their*?" As if coleslaw and bread were owned by the servants.

With that, Mother went into action. Grabbing my brother and me, and with a look at Dad ordering him to follow, she rose from the table, announcing, "Let's get out of here before he comes back."

We were no more than three feet from the table, heading toward the door, when the waiter—"Dad's friend," as mother would later sarcastically call him—reappeared. "Is anything the matter?" he asked with a hurt expression.

With a lame excuse, Dad spoke up, "No, nothing's wrong, buddy. I just forgot my pocketbook." With that, we were out the door.

In the car, Mother turned to Dad and in a cruel way said, "Your *pocketbook*? A *woman's* pocketbook?" Dad was embarrassed. When mother looked back at us, John and I laughed uneasily. "Your *pocketbook*?" she repeated, trying to get a rise out of Dad. When she turned around a second time, John and I could only manage a half-hearted laugh. Dad's confusing his wallet with a woman's pocketbook was funny, but not *that* funny. Mother was about to taunt Dad a third time, when he said in a firm voice, "Damn it, May Elaine, you know I meant wallet!

Damn it! Not in front of the boys!" This was only the second time we had ever heard him curse. Mother became silent.

Mother slept late that Saturday morning because, as she put it, we "owed her that time." In fact, she did every Saturday. While she slept, Dad became someone entirely new, a character very unlike his real-life self. Playfully he would stalk into our rooms, tear the sheets off our bed like a tough guy, and order us to "get dressed and go into the kitchen!" We would pretend to be scared, jumping hastily into our clothes and then racing to the table. Meanwhile, Dad would be cooking breakfast. In that same big iron frying pan he used to roast chestnuts he would throw in eggs, bacon, potatoes, sliced tomatoes, grits, even some leftover spaghetti. All in one pan! Then, when it was cooked, he would bring the frying pan to the table and, scooping out what looked like a large disfigured and discolored pancake, hurl down the food at our plates, all the while faking a scowl, like some mean-spirited short-order cook in a sleazy restaurant. With mock terror, John and I pretended to cower as if, fearing that we weren't showing enough enthusiasm for the ill-shaped mass he had created, we would be beaten like disloyal servants.

"You like this grub?" Dad would bellow.

"Yes, Dad, yes."

"Put a little more life into that 'yes,' boy."

"YES!"

"That's better. You want more grub?"

"Yes, sir."

"Sir? Now that's my boys." He would break into a smile, throw off the stage role, and become once again that sweet, mild-mannered, compassionate man we loved so deeply. John and I would also remove our actors' masks.

Every third Saturday of every month Dad's musician friends would come over to our house to jam. Dad played saxophone in the big bands of the 1920s, '30s, and, for a time, in the '40s. By the 1950s, of course, musical tastes had changed and most of those bands went out of business. When the old men with white hair opened their cases to take out their instruments, a sweet, musty smell filled the air. Trumpets, saxes, trombones, drums, and clarinets filled our living room with "String of Pearls," "Red Sails in the Sunset," "All of Me," "I Only Have Eyes for You," "Up a Lazy River," "Easy Street," "Tuxedo Junction"—songs from a different era. In the style of the Goodman Band, trumpets swayed in unison to the right and then the left, the sax players, including Dad, resting their instruments on their right knee and beating out the rhythm by stamping the floor with the left foot. These old friends played without a conductor, so familiar with each other that a mere wink of the eye became the go-ahead for a solo, the feel, the presence of fellow musicians enough to set the tempo or alter one.

Seeing Dad so vibrant, so accepted, one of the "boys," there on the bandstand before an imaginary audience swinging and swaying, John and I looked at him without Mother's demeaning eyes. One of the men in the band, spotting me, would call out, "Hey, little Sid, come down here, boy, and join us." I lived for such moments. Bounding down the stairs, I would make my way to the piano amid the bottles of Schmidt's beer and the bowls of pretzels littering the room. My job was to bang out chords, to "hit the ivories" as one of the men used to call the keys. I never got to do a solo; I modulated chords as a counterpoint to the drummer's rhythm.

Mother, just barely tolerating the "noise," as she called it, would be in the kitchen, making her own contrapuntal rhythm as she typed a gossip column for *The Breeze*, the local newspaper. The owner paid her by the column inch, and so she banged out reams of copy, no item being too insignificant.

"Mrs. Winer delighted the Martins with a simply delicious Bundt cake last Thursday when the two families gathered for their monthly canasta game."

"Not getting enough of the sand and surf, Mrs. Pace and the children are extending their Ocean City vacation for two days. Poor Freddie, however, has to come back Sunday for the Monday morning shift at the Schmidt's Brewery."

"Little Mildred Bosshart placed fifth in the county spelling bee, and to celebrate the occasion her mother took her to the Casa Argenio Restaurant for a special lunch. Asked about the meal, Mildred said, "Yummy!""

We could hear the peck, peck, peck of that old Lucy Schmidt typewriter long after the last note had died and Dad's friends left.

CHAPTER 8

Being Different

The next time before I went to Charlie's Corner I dropped in on my physician friend John Graham-Pole.

"John, I think I screwed up last Friday. I told the kids a story that had a death at the end."

"You're worried about it?"

"Come on, the last thing the kids need on the Bone Marrow Unit are morbid stories."

"Why?"

"John, you know better than anyone. It's obvious. There's death all around them. They die. Besides, what can I tell them about death?"

"You think that you're intruding on some space sacred to them?

"Yes . . . I guess. I just don't want to add to the problem."

"But they need to face it, Sid, and, actually, your stories ease them into whatever might happen. It's good to remind them of the world outside, a world they might return to, or

at least need to remember. You didn't make a mistake. In fact, you did just the right thing."

"Are you suggesting that—"

A brilliant pediatric oncologist, John also had two revealing, complementary avocations. He was a fine poet and—perhaps even more to the point—was a professional clown. John would sometimes make rounds in clown's makeup, or wear absurdly large floppy shoes. He suggested that I tell them a comic story about death purposely—for my sake as well as theirs.

Sitting by herself some distance from the four boys was a teenage girl. The boys signaled that her being there threatened our "club."

"I'm Amanda," and then she whispered. "They don't want me here."

"We'll deal with that." With the challenge from John Graham-Pole in my mind, I said, "Did I ever tell you the story about **The Black Sheep***?"*

At one Thanksgiving Day dinner Aunt Grace called my Uncle Eddie "the black sheep of the family." "After all," she explained, "he *is* an embarrassment, isn't he?" Well, it was true: Uncle Eddie didn't always act like the rest of us. He didn't even look like us. A big man, with a beer belly and arms like a wrestler's, his face flushed, Uncle Eddie always had a drink in his hand. For most of his life he had worked as a coal miner in upstate Pennsylvania, but finally, urged on by his wife, my Aunt Silvia, they moved to the city and he became a barber.

His barber shop was a man's hangout, located in the living room of their house; Aunt Silvia never set foot in there. Uncle Eddie's customers, all old friends, thought of the shop as their private club. Each had his own shaving mug on the wall. There was a dartboard in the corner. You could even step into a little side room and "draw a brew," as Uncle Eddie used to say. There were also girlie magazines on a table. Uncle Eddie's regulars came not only for a haircut but to talk and visit, and just enjoy each other's company. They stayed for hours, and I remember Aunt Silvia shooing them out when they got in the way of her dinner, which she always served at seven, an hour after the shop was supposed to close.

Uncle Eddie was a rough man, as naturally rough as Aunt Silvia wanted to appear refined. Mother didn't want us to spend time with him; "a bad influence, a boozer" was her assessment. Still, to save money she let Uncle Eddie cut our hair. So, there I would be, getting a crew cut as I listened to the men gossip about the latest neighborhood scandal or saw them duck into that back room for that brew. When Uncle Eddie finished my hair, he would strike a match, one of the long-stemmed ones you use to light wood in a fireplace, and run it all around my head. He said singeing the ends of the hair kept them from splitting. He could have set me on fire, but I trusted Uncle Eddie. Even now I can feel his big left hand holding my head steady as, with his right, he singed the hair, all the while chatting on.

Uncle Eddie gave haircuts to black people, and more than once I saw him kick someone out of the shop for objecting to this. "A head is a head" was his motto; in fact, that motto was right there behind the barber chair, on a little handmade sign dangling from the nose of a moose a taxidermist had given him as a Christmas present. Uncle Eddie lived in a rough section of the city, and though the stores around him were often robbed, no one ever broke into Eddie's. This was partly because everyone in the neighborhood liked him, blacks and whites alike, and partly because Uncle Eddie was known to carry a gun. On the wall was a plaque announcing that he had won the Kiwanis Marksmanship Trophy for the last nine years.

I loved him, even if he was the black sheep. He and Aunt Silvia were childless, and when he called me "Sonny," he'd smile, put that big wrestler's hand around my shoulder, and look down at me paternally.

The black sheep never shocked us so much as at the funeral of his brother Arthur. All of us had gone that afternoon to the parlor in Jenkintown to pay our respects. There was Uncle Arthur in the casket, the top propped up so that everyone could take one last look. Actually, this dead Arthur didn't look much like his real-life self. His once bushy eyebrows were cropped, his hair parted down the middle—Arthur never combed his hair when he was alive—and there was rouge on his cheeks that, Mother said, made him look a bit like a harlot. Mr. Ball, the undertaker, spoke softly about the art of "funereal cosmetics" on "the loved ones." He talked in whispers, as if the dead would wake if anyone used their normal voice. My mother all in black stood in the corner next to Aunt Silvia and Francis, Arthur's wife.

Every once in a while you could hear a bit of conversation. "He was a good man, that he was." "Well, he's gone to a finer place than this, that's for sure." "They say he died peacefully." "Why Arthur? The man was a saint." I was thirteen at the time, and didn't know much about death, but it seemed funny to hear all these nice things being said about Arthur because, as I recall, nobody had said anything good about Arthur when he was alive. Especially not Aunt Francis. Now here they were, reminding each other how "wonderful" he was, how much they'd miss him. Aunt Francis constantly dabbed a little pink hanky to her right eye. Every few minutes, someone would walk over to the casket, let out a deep sigh, loud enough so that the people talking would turn in their direction, nod with approval, and then fall to murmuring again. Mr. Ball stood in the far corner, pleased with himself; his wife made the rounds of the guests with a little silver tray overflowing with heart-shaped pieces of cheese and watercress sandwiches.

Suddenly Uncle Eddie showed up. He was drunk. Pushing aside the double doors at the far end of the room, he clung to them, his big body filling the entire entrance. His face was very red. "Oh no, he's been drinking!" someone whispered. Another confirmed the judgment with an "again"; a third added, "Imagine, at his own brother's funeral!"

Spotting the casket at the far end, Uncle Eddie moaned "Arthur" loudly and started to cross towards it. As he weaved among them, people parted as if he had some contagious disease. Aunt Francis turned very pale and began to wipe her forehead with the pink hanky. Mother made a loud "Ahem" in her throat, to send her brother a sign she disapproved.

Uncle Eddie was now halfway towards the casket, and there wasn't a sound in the room. He was walking in a wobbly way, as if his feet weren't sure the floor was there to support him. I was afraid he would fall. Then he stopped, searched through the crowd and, spotting me, called out, "Give me a hand, little Sid." Too late my mother hissed "No" at me as Uncle Eddie's big hand reached out and he wrapped it around my shoulder, using me as a sort of crutch. "Help me to Arthur, Sid?" he crooned in a sad half-whisper, the words all slurred. We made our way to Arthur.

As everyone else looked on in horror, he cried, "Pray with me?" We knelt down together beside the casket. I couldn't make out what Uncle Eddie was saying, but big tears were falling down his cheeks, followed by a sob deep inside his chest. Soon, his whole chest was pumping up and down; the sobbing pervaded the room. Some people gasped, a few others laughed. Uncle Eddie must have heard this because he bolted up, turned toward the crowd, and in his big, bass voice cried out, "I loved him. I *loved* him . . . you bunch of dried-up old maggots!"

"Well of all the—" someone exclaimed, but never finished the sentence.

Uncle Eddie was now looking down at his brother, gesturing with his hands towards the dead man, as if he were trying to communicate with him in sign language. Words would start to come but then were choked off. Suddenly, he put his big arm on the far side of the coffin and, in an instant, pole-vaulted himself right into the box, so that he was now lying face to face with Arthur. Beside a dead man!

"Arthur, oh, Arthur, it's me, Eddie! Arthur, I love you so much!"

Behind me I heard people say things like "Disgusting!" and "What did you expect?" and "This time he's gone too far!" There was a noise from the side, and I turned to see people gathering around Aunt Francis: She had fainted. My mother stormed out of the room. In a few seconds, Dad and some of the other men came over and, with a little resistance from Uncle Eddie—in fact, with a *lot* of resistance—pulled him out of the casket.

Given what had happened, it was decided that my parents and I would spend that night with Aunt Silvia. "Who knows what that madman might do?" Mother told Dad in the car. After seeing to Aunt Silvia, who, very upset, kept repeating "How humiliating . . . how humiliating" as she climbed the stairs to the second floor, my parents made me a bed on the living room sofa and then went upstairs to the spare room. Uncle Eddie had to sleep in the car, outside in the alley behind their row house. This was where he slept anytime he got drunk. A sort of punishment, or an exile, you might say. Aunt Silvia always forgave him in a day or two, but until she did the car was where he slept.

I tossed and turned, and couldn't get out of my mind those big tears I had seen fall from Uncle Eddie's eyes. Nor that deep sob. And how he had called the mourners "dried-up old maggots." I chuckled at that. Now, I know you're supposed to be quiet and dignified at funerals, paying your respects to the dead and all that. My mother had called what Uncle Eddie did "the most despicable thing" she had ever seen. Still, he did love his brother, loved him so much that he had leaped right into the casket. Right beside a dead man! Yet I think I understood. I loved my brother John, even though we fought a lot. In a way, what Uncle Eddie did seemed *beautiful.* Beautiful. That's the only word that came to me.

I got out of bed, put on my bathrobe, and sneaked back to the kitchen. In an instant, I had opened the back door and was making my way to the car. There was Uncle Eddie, sound asleep in the back seat, curled up like a little baby, an empty bottle in his big hand. The air was getting cold, so I went back to the house, found a blanket in the hall linen closet, and returned to the car. I pulled the blanket up and around Uncle Eddie, just the way my dad used to do for me. He stirred slightly, tried to lift his head, mumbled something, and fell back to sleep. Whatever he had done or hadn't done, the black sheep was at peace in his world.

"The Black Sheep" got the usual critical review. The boys fixed on the moment when my uncle pole-vaulted into the coffin. Freddie reminded us that "your body gets real cold when you're dead."

All this time Amanda remained silent, but not uninterested. She sat there all by herself, still convinced that the boys hated her.

"Why don't you boys invite Amanda to sit over here?"

"She's a girl!"

"She's different."

"Different?"

"Yeah," James said

Finally, Tommy spoke. "Amanda, you wanna come over here?"

Amanda got up slowly when Freddie moved a seat to one side. She hurried to it.

"So, now can we have our second story?"

"Now that you boys have put some sense in your head, yes."

"Did I ever tell you a story called **They Never Asked Me***?"*

"Say 'no,'" Freddie told her, a bit roughly, awkwardly.

Amanda let out a clear soprano "No."

⁓☆⁓

Richard Fasser was quiet, *very* quiet. He never spoke. If you asked his opinion, or even just said something to him, he'd only smile, without saying a word. If you pressed him for a "yes" or "no," he would smile, give a simple nod, but nothing more. Richard did all his work in class; he was a good student and we all knew this because one day, by mistake, the teacher mixed up Arlene Cake's report card with his, and Arlene later told us that Richard got all A's. Yet teachers never called on him in class, and, of course, Richard never put his hand up to give an answer or ask a question. One of the busybody mothers once pressed Miss McFeeney, the principal, on why Richard didn't have to answer the teachers' questions like the rest of us. She was abruptly told that this was "school policy with Richard."

Richard looked like a nobody. There was nothing distinct, nothing special about his features. It was as if nature had taken the average of boys his age and come up with the most inconspicuous of people. Still, there was something comforting about him, for he remained quiet and impassive to a degree that I suspected life's tragedies as well as comedies would pass him by.

Our nickname for him was "The Stone." We never called him that to his face because everyone liked Richard, even though none of us had ever really spoken to him or—to be more accurate—had ever known him to speak to us, beyond that occasional "yes" or "no" or a smile which seemed to say he had heard what we said, was thinking about it, but had nothing to say in return. Yes, everyone liked Richard because even though he was the "The Stone" of Cedar Road Elementary School, he was also the most polite of our classmates. If Richard was waiting in line in front of you and you tapped him on the shoulder, he'd turn around when you said, "Hi, Richard," though, of course, he wouldn't say "Hi" back. You could count on that. Yet right there on the spot, he would get behind you so you could take his place. Break a pencil and Richard gave you one of his own. One day, just as we were going to Gym, I asked Karen Litz, who sat behind me, if I could borrow some notebook paper for Spelling, which came right after Gym. Karen, who was stingy, shook her head "no." The bell rang, and I figured that, when we got back to class, I would simply ask someone else. When I returned from Gym, however, there were ten brand-new sheets of paper on my desk. I looked over at Richard. When I said "thank you," he smiled that smile. If I had said, "Did you do this?" he might have said "yes" but nothing more.

A mystery—a mystery of silence. Everyone had a different idea why. The Rupert brothers, who always agreed with each other, said that their mother told them Richard had a "lazy tongue." They weren't sure just what a lazy tongue was, but since the Rupert brothers always agreed with their mother, they said it must be so. "Maybe he's just real shy—I mean *real* shy," Barbara Pace suggested. Nancy Holloway figured Richard must be a genius, with the brain of a thirty-year-old man, and so all us other kids seemed dumb to him. Jimmy Neil suspected Richard had suffered a tragedy, like seeing his father die, and silence was the result, Richard's way of avoiding the world where all the rest of us—well, almost all the rest of us—had fathers. When someone pointed out to Jimmy that Richard's father was alive, Jimmy got angry and hit back with, "OK, maybe it was his grandfather! You ever seen him alive?" Miyo, our exchange student from Japan, pictured Richard as the Buddha, yet that idea only confused us more. Many kids thought Richard had some dark secret weighing on him like a heavy stone. Alison Price, already writing poetry, claimed that Richard "lived inside himself." "Why don't you just ask him why he's so quiet?" Megan Hanrahan suggested, but I told her that if you did, Richard would probably just smile unless you said, "Are you quiet because of so and so?" You'd have to put some reason in place of the "so and so" and force a "yes" or "no" out of Richard. The next day Megan tried it, and when we asked her what happened, she said that instead of an answer one way or the other, Richard just smiled.

Some of us asked our sixth-grade teacher, Mrs. Belsky, about Richard. We all loved Mrs. Belsky; she was the one teacher we could talk to about such things. She said there was a reason Richard was so silent but that she could not us tell us. David Salisbury asked, "When you say 'I cannot tell you,' does that mean you don't want to tell us, or that you don't know?" Mrs. Belsky smiled, "That's for me to know and you to find out." Then she patted David on the head and told him she had papers to grade.

So that's how it was. Richard was silent and just why remained a mystery. There's no denying he was polite and we all liked him. He came to school, said nothing all day, and went right home. I liked Alison's idea, that Richard "lived inside himself," but that didn't tell me or anybody else *why*. Or what it was like to be that way. Or if he liked being that way, *if* he was that way. You certainly couldn't ask Richard why he lived inside himself.

Then one day everything changed.

Normally I went to Ormandy's grocery for my mother about three in the afternoon. Ormandy's was one of those old-fashioned stores, before there were supermarkets. You didn't pick things off the shelf but instead went to the counter and told Mr. Ormandy what you wanted, or you'd give him a list. He'd get everything for you since almost all the cans and boxes were on high shelves behind the counter. Mr. Ormandy's store was actually the front room of his house, and right behind the counter, surrounded by shelves, was a door. It was always half-open, and the thing to do, while Mr. Ormandy went about getting your order, was to peek through the opening and look into the second room. Sometimes, you could see his daughter sitting in a big wingback chair. She never came into the store; she always stayed in that room behind the counter. Mother said that there was "something wrong" with the Ormandy girl, that she was crazy—my mother used the phrase "mentally ill"—or retarded, or possibly a little bit of both. We never met a Mrs. Ormandy. No one ever saw the daughter clearly, or for long, although one time, while Mr. Ormandy was getting something from the front of the store, Bruzzy Fleck tried to sneak around the counter to get a better look. Mr. Ormandy spotted him and ordered Bruzzy out of the store. He was never allowed to shop at Ormandy's again.

I had glimpsed the daughter many times. She had short, cropped hair, and strange eyes that seemed to bulge. She was thin, and very pale. It was hard to tell just how old she was. People guessed anywhere from twenty to forty.

No one knew much about Mr. Ormandy either. He was always courteous, talking about the weather or once in a while commenting on something that happened in the neighborhood. He actually spoke very little, and usually the moment you had paid, he'd say good-bye in a way that meant it was time for you to leave.

It was a little scary going to Ormandy's—the idea of that girl in the room behind the counter, never coming out, never speaking. We'd see Mr. Ormandy on the street now and then, but without his daughter. For all we knew, she'd never been outside.

"Maybe she was born in that room and that's where she'll die," I heard Mr. Klecto say to my father when they were having their regular Saturday chat over the back fence. Some kids predicted if the Ormandy girl was crazy, one day while you were at the counter she just might come charging out with a butcher knife and try to stab you. I heard one mother suggest that maybe she's wasn't Mr. Ormandy's daughter at all but his prisoner. Or maybe his "child bride." Then, one day all this speculation about the Ormandy girl took a new turn. And Richard Fasser was involved.

Running out of flour just as she was about to make dinner, my mother told me to go down to Ormandy's before it closed at six. When I got there, Richard was waiting at the counter. Mr. Ormandy was at the front of the store getting his order. I had never seen Richard any place but at school. While Mr. Ormandy was busy, I walked up to Richard.

"How ya doing?"

Richard just smiled.

I tried again. "You usually come here around this time?"

He smiled and then said "yes."

"I usually come at three but my mother ran out of flour so that's why I'm here now." I felt like an idiot. I mean, what did it matter when I came to Ormandy's?

Richard smiled, as if he understood.

Just then we saw her, the Ormandy girl! This time she wasn't sitting in the chair. No, she stood right there in the doorway. On every other occasion I had seen just a bit of her, and then only for a second, but now I could see her from head to toe, and for more than a second. She stood there in the doorway, looking at us. Her hair was awfully short, but it was a soft brown color, and while she was thin and pale, somehow she looked like the beautiful ivory statue of the Virgin Mary on my Aunt Grace's bureau. She seemed both young and old, or as if she were young on the outside but old inside. There she stood, staring straight ahead, not rudely, just staring. Richard and I exchanged glances. When Mr. Ormandy climbed down the ladder with Richard's order and we turned back to the counter, she was gone.

I was so shocked by what had just happened that, after Richard paid for his groceries, I forgot all about getting the flour and instead walked out of the store with him.

We looked at each other. Forgetting that Richard never spoke except to say "yes" or "no," I asked, "I wonder what it's like spending all your life in that room?"

"I've been wondering the same thing."

Not realizing at first that Richard had actually said something more than his usual "yes" or "no," I continued, "I hope she's happy."

From somewhere deep inside, almost as if he were praying, I heard him reply, "I hope so too, Sid."

With that, Richard walked down the street without looking back. I stood there dumbfounded that he had spoken to me. Two simple sentences—"I've been wondering the same thing" and "I hope so too, Sid"—but just now they seemed a book-full of words, *volumes*.

There was another surprise the following afternoon. Richard's mother called our house at lunch time, saying her son had invited me to come home from school with him the next day and play until dinner. The following morning when I told the other kids at school, at first no one would believe me. Later, the invitation sank in, especially after I told everyone the two miraculous things that had happened, about seeing the Ormandy girl in the doorway and then actually talking with Richard outside the store. My friends became detectives, going over our conversation with microscopes, making connections between Richard and the Ormandy girl, even saying it was fate that made my mother run out of flour so that I would go to the store while Richard was there.

That afternoon, as Richard and I walked out of the school and across the playground on our way to his home, our classmates stepped to the side, giving us room as if I were passing with Moses through the Red Sea.

I had a wonderful time at Richard's house. After we checked in with his mother, we went to the backyard, which was bisected by a swift-flowing stream. Richard, as usual, said very little, almost nothing. We communicated by some inner sense. First we dammed up the stream, using bricks that had been stacked behind the house, then plugged the gaps with thick mud from the banks. It was the best dam I'd ever built. Within a half-hour the stream had grown into a small pond. From his father's toolshed we dragged out an old raft, pushed it into the pond, and sailed around in circles, using two poles left over from a volleyball set as oars.

At four Mrs. Fasser called us for a snack. She served iced tea laced with mint and the most delicious chocolate-chip cookies I had ever eaten. Mrs. Fasser was beautiful. Tall, with jet black hair, she moved about the kitchen like some graceful animal, like a deer. It was clear that she loved Richard, just by the way she put her hand on his shoulder, or gently placed an extra cookie on his plate. Like Richard, she said very little. The house itself was a quiet place. A clock ticked effortlessly on the wall.

After our snack we went into the living room to play cards. I had never seen a place like this. There were paintings on the walls, a mixture of modern and classic artists, arranged in such a way that from time to time I let my eyes wander back and forth among them, as if they were flowers in a bouquet. Two sofas covered in dark leather faced each other at angles before the fireplace, and the large bay windows on the opposite side of the room were framed with deep red velvet curtains. I felt as if I were on a movie set, or in a time far removed from the one I knew. There was a sophistication about this room; everything, from the furniture to the hardwood floor, was elegant and understated. I could imagine Richard, with his parents, sitting here at night, before the fire, surrounded by those paintings, sipping tea with mint leaves—all saying very little.

It was so quiet you could even hear the sounds of our cards, not just when they were shuffled but as we discarded or picked one from the pile. As always, Richard remained silent, and yet I felt relaxed, at peace with him.

At five Mrs. Fasser came in to tell me it was time to go home. She thanked me for coming. Richard himself said nothing, although he smiled as I left. Still, that smile was different from the one he usually gave at school, in a way that I could not measure. Halfway down the street I turned to look at his house. Richard was in the backyard, tearing the dam apart. Why would he do this? In a few minutes the stream subsided, and then I saw him walk towards the back door, just as his father's car pulled into the driveway. A moment later, Richard and Mrs. Fasser came out the front door. All three were standing very close together, and Mr. Fasser had put his arms around them.

The next day Richard returned to his old self, as if I had only dreamed that conversation outside Ormandy's store or gone to his house. Wordless yet as polite as ever, Richard treated me with the same benign silence, perhaps even indifference as he did everyone else. Things were back to normal. I never received another invitation to play at Richard's house. But somehow, in a way I can't express even to myself, I think I understood him. When friends asked me what it was like to be at his house, I borrowed Mrs. Belsky's expression, "That's for me to know and you to find out."

Things stayed as usual with Richard until three months later when the Ormandy's store was robbed. Richard was involved. The paper reported that a robber had entered Ormandy's at six, just as it was about to close. Richard was the sole customer. The robber had forced Mr. Ormandy and Richard into that living room behind the counter and tied them up, along with Mr. Ormandy's daughter. Imagine, Richard had even been in the same room with her! A few hours after the robber left, Richard managed to get himself untied, but—now here's the crazy thing—once he was free he picked up the groceries he had bought and walked out of the store; he left Mr. Ormandy and his daughter still tied up. When Richard got home he said nothing to his parents about the robbery! Early the next morning a deliveryman heard the Ormandys crying for help. When the robber was caught two days later, Richard went with his parents to the police station to help identify him. According to the paper, when the police asked Richard why he hadn't untied the Ormandys, he simply replied, "I had to go home." When questioned why he hadn't told his parents, he said, "They never asked me."

For a few weeks Richard's two answers became a running joke in school. A kid would come up to you and say something like, "Why did you let those twenty people get run over by a garbage truck?" You were supposed to answer, "I had to go home." Or, "Why didn't you tell your parents you won a million dollars?" and of course you'd say, "They never asked me." When Richard overheard the kids making these jokes about him, he just smiled—and said nothing. I think I can understand why.

Like some of my characters, I myself was "different" as a child, a mother's boy who was never really popular in school, awkward with girls, dismal at sports. I was an outsider, like Amanda, Richard Fasser, and even Mr. Ormandy's daughter. I realized I had chosen the story about Richard Fasser that day because the boys had treated Amanda like someone different. But I knew Amanda and Tommy had really listened when I heard him say to her, "Don't worry. It doesn't hurt

when they shave your head." James added, "They nicked me
when they did it but . . . no . . . he's right, it doesn't hurt."

To reward them, on my next visit I would tell them about
The Queen of the Mushrooms.

⟿⟐⟿

Dick Robino and his sister Marie were what we called
"bookends"—opposites. They looked alike but were as different as day and night.

Marie was pretty but plump, her face covered with freckles,
her hair a striking red. She had asthma and whenever the class
was quiet you could hear her breath. I tried to imagine what
Marie would look like if she were thinner and didn't have all
those freckles. Would they disappear with time?

Each morning when Marie got to class she would take four
pencils from a little box and then ask the teacher's permission
to sharpen them. Once they were sharpened, she'd arrange
them parallel to each other in the upper-right-hand corner of
her desk, *always* in the upper-right-hand corner. Next she
would find one of those circular erasers, attached to a brush,
and very carefully remove any little black threads that came
from using it. However, instead of dropping the threads on the
floor as the rest of us might have done, Marie would put them
in the palm of her right hand, raise her left, and ask the teacher
permission to discard the threads in the wastebasket near the
front desk. Marie would never have thought of dropping the
threads on the floor. Finally, she would take five sheets of white

paper—not four, not six, but five, *always* five—and place them in the exact center of her desk. Once this was done, she would quietly fold her hands and wait for class to begin.

Marie Robino was the most generous person I had ever known. At lunch, if she had a package of Tastycakes, and there were three people at her table who wanted one, she would give away all three. If you said to her, "Why don't you save one for yourself, Marie?" she would reply, "No thank you. That's just fine." Everything was always "just fine" with Marie. If you were at the water fountain, she would leave whatever she was doing and turn on the spigot for you. If there was one child too many for the seats on a school bus, she would volunteer to stand.

However appealing her modesty may have been, there was one problem with Marie. She was dull.

Now her brother Dick was a different case. He had an opinion about everything, and he could talk you into anything. A big guy, fat like his sister, somehow his fatness made him seem manly, or at least fearsome. Dick had the same red hair and freckles. There was something "bad" about him, a bit of the devil, and that just made him more fascinating.

In seventh grade, for example, Dick played a great trick on Miss Framer, our homeroom teacher. Afraid of becoming an "old maid," she tried to do everything to make herself attractive. We suspected she had a crush on Mr. Kelly, the good-looking biology teacher. Miss Framer wasn't very attractive, and the most awful thing about her were her glasses. She had to wear thick, owl-like lenses, but she was always taking them off because she knew she looked worse with them on.

One day when Miss Framer was sitting at her desk without her glasses on, Dick Robino took a spool of very thin (but very strong) fishing line and tied it to the leg of his desk. Then, he had the rest of us pass the line back and forth between the first two rows, weaving it like a spider's web around the desk legs, up and down the two rows, back and forth. When we were finished, it looked like some crazy version of Cat's Cradle, resting just a half-foot or so above the floor.

Dick went to the back of the room and, right there, lit a cigarette. Without her glasses on, Miss Framer saw him only as a blur, but she could sure smell tobacco burning.

"Who's smoking a cigarette?" she shouted, still not putting on her glasses.

"I am, Miss Framer. What you gonna do about it?" Dick sassed back.

"Richard Robino, stop that at once!"

"Come and make me, 'teach'!"

With an incredulous "Why you!—" Miss Framer got up and started down the row. She hadn't gone more than a few feet when she became hopelessly entangled in "Robino's Web." The more she struggled, the more she got caught. Soon she was pitching back and forth, like a big ship rocking in the waves. Dick was laughing his head off; kids up and down the rows were betting how long she could keep her balance. Now she was thrashing about, her hands sawing the air. In a few seconds Miss Framer started shrieking the way a wounded elephant does or a mouse caught in a trap, and then she toppled right over, encased in fishing line, like an Egyptian mummy entombed right there between the desks.

At that very moment Dr. Poole, the principal, came through the door. "What . . . what's going on here?"

From the back Dick Robino volunteered, "I don't know what's happened to Miss Framer, Dr. Poole. She's just not herself today."

The class exploded into laughter. Dr. Poole told some of us to get Miss Framer untangled. She raced from the room in tears. We had a substitute the rest of the day. As for Dick Robino, he was suspended for two weeks, and when he returned, he was the most popular boy in school. It was fun to embarrass Miss Framer like that. After all, if she had worn her glasses none of this would have happened. Still, I myself couldn't or wouldn't do what Dick Robino did. He certainly was interesting, as interesting as his sister Marie was dull.

That's why my brother and I were so excited when Dick asked us one day at school to come over to his house that afternoon. Actually, he didn't exactly ask me if we'd like to come, but rather said something like, "You can come over with John this afternoon." An odd way to invite someone. Still, I was so eager to go I didn't care.

Dick's mom showed us toward his bedroom. He was sitting on the floor, surrounded by packets of postage stamps, with a large album between his legs. He didn't say hello when he saw us but only motioned for us to sit on the floor.

"I've got every stamp ever printed in the United States," he said proudly. No word that he was glad to see us.

"Every stamp?" John asked with more than a touch of doubt in his voice.

I was a little embarrassed by my brother because his question sounded too much like a challenge, and I very much wanted to be a friend of Dick Robino. Imagine what the kids at school would say if I were known as his buddy!

"Every stamp," Dick replied.

Just as coolly, John shot back, "*Every* stamp?"

"What goes with this little punk?" Dick said, looking at me.

I gave him a you-know-how-little-brothers-can-be expression. John saw it too. His head, lowered for a second, told me I had hurt him.

However, when John looked back up, straight at Dick Robino, there was fire in his eyes.

"Well, I don't think you have *every* stamp. I mean, nobody has *every* stamp."

"I do so!"

"OK. Do you have the 13-cent air-mail stamp with a picture of Washington crossing the Delaware?"

"Sure."

"What about the 25-cent blue one with the 'Spirit of Saint Louis'?"

"Of course!"

"The 5-cent Jefferson one-day issue, in brown instead of the green that's more common?"

"Yeah."

"I bet you don't have the dollar one with the double picture of the soldier and sailor?"

"I do, too!"

It went on like this for ten minutes. Dick had every stamp John mentioned. He never bothered to prove it to us, but then John didn't ask for proof. The two were sparring, stamp-crazed boxers circling the ring. John jabbed: "The post-due stamp used just on federal mail? The one with Betsy Ross sewing the American flag?" Dick punched back with "Sure" and "Of course." He looked so confident. John looked confident. Dick was clearly annoyed.

John was soaring. He didn't look like a punk now, and I began to regret that look I had given Dick earlier when he had called him one. For his part Dick no longer seemed so glamorous. John renewed the attack, and this time there was a malevolent joy in his voice.

"Do you have that 20-cent stamp with the picture of a man wrestling a pig?"

"Of course!"

"How about that 2 1/2-cent stamp from the 1870s that shows a baby sucking his thumb?"

Acting as if to hesitate were to lose, or like a cat with his back against the wall, Dick blurted out, "Yeah, sure I do."

Then John delivered the final punch. "And what about that joint issue of Mexico and the U.S. showing a cowboy eating from a can of beans? It's very rare."

"Yes, yes, *yes* I do!!!" Dick screamed, pounding the floor with his fist.

"You damn fool! You stupid idiot," John said slowly, full of contempt. "There are no such stamps. I just made up the one about the pig wrestling and the baby sucking his thumb. And you . . . *you* idiot . . . you fell for the one about the cowboy! A can of beans?—you liar!"

"You, little punk, think you can make a fool of me? You know who I am? Dick Robino! Dick Robino! I'm Dick Robino. I've got the best stamp collection in town—maybe the state. You stupid little . . . ! Get out of my room! Out of my room! You tricked me!"

Mrs. Robino came running in and, taking one look at her son, said, "I think you owe your guests an apology, Richard." Alternately sobbing, screaming, and cursing, Dick rushed into the bathroom, slamming the door.

His mother looked as if she wanted to explain, but, embarrassed for her sake, John and I thanked her for having us over and quickly made our way out.

By mistake, we took the back door instead of the front. We didn't care—John was triumphant. I was so proud of him. There, standing in the far corner of the yard, was Marie. My head was spinning from what had just happened. You know, sometimes you just have to trust your impulses. Pushing John by the arm, I walked over to Marie and said "Hi."

At least *Marie* seemed pleased to see us. Impulse struck again. Right there, as if the words came to me without thinking, as if by magic, I said to her, "Marie, can you tell me something interesting, *really* interesting that *you* do?'

No sooner had I said this than I began to regret it. After all, this was the dull Marie Robino, the girl with no personality, the girl who took her erasure shavings up to the teacher's wastebasket instead of flicking them on the floor.

Unexpectedly, Marie spoke in a voice so clear, so strong that John and I couldn't believe our ears.

"Yes, I can." Then she added, in a very polite way, as if there were a "please" before and after her "Come on."

She took us across the yard to a big mound of earth with a door in it, leading into a storm cellar.

"Would you like to see my mushroom collection?"

Mushroom collection? Still in a state of shock, John and I said "yes" together. Opening the door and turning on a light, Marie led us down eight steps into a damp room with a strange sweet smell.

Before us were millions of mushrooms—brown, green, white, purple, multicolored. In every shape you could imagine—clouds, cones, saucers, spaceships, cubes. Row after row, villages, towns, cities, states of mushrooms hiding there in the darkened room. I was especially taken by a large clump of tall white mushrooms that, all together, looked like skyscrapers lining a city block. Marie moved like a queen among her subjects, identifying mushrooms first by their Latin and then their English names, telling us how they grew, about mushrooms in history, and what famous people had said about mushrooms. I never heard her speak so much, nor so eloquently. And while I can't ever imagine myself taking mushrooms that seriously, still, she made them seem fascinating.

Marie told us her father had written articles about mushrooms in scientific journals; she had learned the hobby from him.

She touched the mushrooms as if they were diamonds. Here was Marie Robino, Queen of the Mushrooms, in a kingdom of dim light, suffused with the cool, sweet, musty smell of mushrooms, her kingdom below the surface, hidden and unknown.

After an hour or so, we finally heard Mrs. Robino calling Marie for dinner. As we came back through the double doors leading to the backyard, even though the sun had gone down, the twilight blinded us. Looking towards the second floor of the house we could see Dick, still pacing about in his room, absurdly tracing a circle like one of those mechanical ducks in a shooting gallery. He didn't seem that special anymore, but I knew that there was a special side to his sister, Marie Robino, Queen of the Mushrooms.

CHAPTER 9

Something Good from Something Bad

We live in more than one world at a time; we live in many. Charlie's Corner had become one of those worlds, with its own population, its own customs, its own reason for being. I felt very close to Tommy, to his three teenage friends, and now to Amanda, who was its newest official citizen.

This day in Charlie's Corner the children seemed quieter than usual. I knew from Dr. Graham-Pole that most of them were now in an advanced stage of treatment—harder, more invasive, and more dangerous.

I thought I could help the situation with a few words of encouragement, something about the relation between the pain of treatment and the possibility of a cure, or at least some relief from their suffering, but my words were too abstract and fell flat. I was a foreigner, someone who could talk about their pain but, when all is said and done, an outsider who didn't know what they were going through.

"You wouldn't change places with us for all the money in the world, would you?" one of the teenagers observed, his tone more resigned than combative.

I tried to answer, if indeed I could have answered. But I had no voice; my actor's voice of which I was so proud, which I loved to use at the drop of a hat, my "instrument," as we call it in the theatre, stuck in my throat—was mute.

The ever-polite Grant, seeing my discomfort, came to my rescue. "How about a story where something good comes out of something bad?" Released, relieved, I gladly responded, "Sure. Sure. Let me tell you about **Bruzzy the Bully***."*

We never argued with my mother because she always won. I heard my father argue with her only a few times, and she always won. Except once. That was the time my mother started to walk away, then turned around to add, "Well, Sid, that's just the other side of the same coin." Dad's was at best a partial victory. Still, the phrase stuck in my head—the other side of the same coin. Then I thought about Bruzzy Fleck.

Bruzzy was the classic bully. He never picked on anyone his own size; he beat up on younger, smaller kids. In the winter, when they blocked off the street that ran by his house so we could go sledding, Bruzzy would come flying across from the side, just as we reached the halfway point on the hill, smashing into us with his sled, cutting right in front of us and, with one blow from his big hand, pushing us off. As we tumbled down the hill, he would let out a cruel laugh.

Bruzzy had a big angry face, blotchy skin, and no neck. He used to jam kids inside their lockers—"Bruzzy's prison" he called it. Once Jimmy Neil was stuck there an entire day. On Halloween, Bruzzy scared young children, forcing them to give over all the candy they had collected.

Bruzzy Fleck was a bully; we all hated him. Some said his father beat him, some said his mother drank. I don't know. All I know is that Bruzzy Fleck was a bully, and so you might ask: How could there be two sides to *this* coin?

Bruzzy was especially cruel to Jackie Klineman. Now Jackie was an odd kid. There was something wrong with him. He had a tiny little body, oddly shaped; his arms and legs seemed to have a will of their own. Jackie must have had polio, or some disease like that. Most of the kids called him "voodoo doll" because his face was shrunken like a prune, the skin very dry, and though Jackie was the same age as the rest of us—twelve or thirteen—he looked like an old man. He never spoke. Everyone else carried their books, but Jackie waited for the bus with a satchel tucked under his arm, standing alone under a tree to the left of the cement square where the rest of us used to play games while waiting. Jackie always got on last. One day, when the only seat left was beside Bruzzy Fleck, Jackie tried to stand but the bus driver told him he couldn't. When Jackie started to sit beside him, Bruzzy stretched out so that there was just a little space left on the edge of the seat by the aisle. As Jackie looked down, Bruzzy, in a real loud voice, dared him, "Go 'head, Klineman, there's two inches. Enjoy yourself." Jackie did his best to stay seated, but as the bus jerked around corners, he kept falling to the floor between the rows. Every time he did, Bruzzy broke into that insanely wicked laugh.

From that day on, Bruzzy continually humiliated Jackie. He flicked his fingers against Jackie's ears, which already stood out from his head. He tripped him, or came up behind him giving him wedgies. Sometimes he made fun of the way Jackie walked, or stood there shouting "voodoo doll" at him. He pinched him, stole his satchel, scattered his school papers all around. Bruzzy did just what you'd expect a bully to do, yet somehow with Jackie it was worse. We all wanted to do something; enough was enough. Yet we were afraid. Maybe the situation was funny at first, big Bruzzy and little Jackie. Even repeating Bruzzy's "There's two inches. Enjoy yourself." After a while, though, it wasn't funny. Yet none of us lifted a finger.

We never heard a complaint from Jackie.

That is, until the last day of school. Bruzzy was picking on Jackie as usual, while the rest of us stood by. The bus wasn't due for ten minutes, and on this particular morning Bruzzy especially seemed to enjoy terrorizing Jackie. He stopped only long enough to go over to the water fountain.

Then, while Bruzzy was bent over taking a drink, it happened. We heard coming from Jackie, from deep down in his throat, a sort of gurgling, or maybe it was more like a purring, as if something had gotten caught way down there and he was trying to get it out. The sound got louder and more savage; even Bruzzy turned to look. Soon it was as if all the anger, all the tortures Jackie had suffered in silence from Bruzzy, everything that had been building and building had suddenly found a voice. Jackie's weird sound was not of this earth.

As Bruzzy stood, not moving, mesmerized, the sound stopped as suddenly as it had started. Slowly, his legs and arms going in contrary directions, Jackie walked toward his satchel. The rest of us froze. He put his bony fingers inside. What was in there? He pulled out a pair of scissors and then raised them in the air so that they were pointing directly at Bruzzy. In a few seconds that gurgling returned; this time it was rapid and grating.

Suddenly, Jackie raced toward Bruzzy, the scissors stabbing at the air in front of him. Bruzzy ran, but Jackie was right behind, right on his heels, gurgling and purring, gurgling and purring, those scissors sometimes coming within inches of Bruzzy. Around trees, back and forth over the concrete waiting place, darting among us, like a monster in a horror movie, Jackie pursued Bruzzy.

The bus came just in time. Two seconds later and who knew what would have happened.

"Bruzzy would be there dead on the ground, those scissors quivering in his back, blood gushing out all over," Peggy Schantz predicted.

This time when we got on the bus, Bruzzy, who always used to sit in the back, sat right behind the driver. Jackie took Bruzzy's old seat in back, and though he didn't talk, we did notice that for the first time he calmly read a book.

Next fall, when school started up, we waited for the bus as we always did; Jackie stood beneath the tree. A few times

Bruzzy tried to approach him, but when he did, we would hear—more important, *Bruzzy* would hear—that little gurgling start from Jackie's throat. Bruzzy never bothered Jackie after that. Of course, he did bother us, ditching our sleds, stealing Halloween candy. We were all still scared of Bruzzy, yet maybe not quite so much now.

Mother had said a coin has two sides, and there came a time when by doing something bad Bruzzy actually did something good.

Roy Grittle. We never, ever called him Roy; he was always "Fingers"—Fingers Grittle. For good reason. Ever since he went to Mrs. McMann's kindergarten, ever since we knew him, Roy sucked his fingers. The two forefingers of his right hand were constantly in his mouth; the other hand twirled his cowlick. He did this all the time, without stopping—in class, while talking, at lunch as he chewed his food, on the playground. Alfie Winer once spent the night at Fingers' house and said he did it in his sleep. Fingers' finger sucking was especially embarrassing for Mrs. Grittle. She was a "go-getter," according to my mother, one of those people who get overly involved in community activities. Mrs. Grittle was the president of the PTA, and you should have seen her face the night the PTA's program chairwoman—*my* mother—invited an expert to speak on "Bedwetting and Thumb Sucking: Two Crises for Parents of Elementary School Children."

Nothing could stop Fingers from sucking. With permission from his mother, teachers used to punish him. One year he arrived in class with a special glove on his right hand, which he immediately tried to take off so he could continue sucking those two fingers. Later he claimed he lost the glove. In third grade the doctor put some foul-tasting juice on his hand, but Fingers just sucked it right off. We were even allowed to make fun of him, and sometimes we'd do this by having the whole class pretend to be Fingers, two fingers in our mouths, and the other hand twirling our cowlicks. As a last resort Fingers went to see what my dad called "a mind doctor." Mrs. Grittle even asked my mother for the telephone number of that PTA speaker.

Nothing could stop Fingers from sucking. He'd try to stop, but pretty soon there he'd be back sucking and twirling, twirling and sucking. In junior high school, Nancy Holloway, the prettiest girl in our class, even said she'd go on a date with him *if* he'd stop sucking his fingers. This was a big sacrifice on Nancy's part because Fingers was not especially good looking: gangly, his face pimply, with hair hanging down in wisps over his forehead, as he sucked away he looked like one of those mutant babies we were warned atomic radiation might produce.

"The only things in this life you can be sure of are death, taxes, and that Grittle boy sucking his fingers," Mother once told Mrs. Neil while playing canasta.

In junior high school it really got embarrassing, not so much for Fingers, who just kept sucking away anyway, as for the rest of us. In Social Studies you'd hear that telltale slurp, slurp, slurp in the back row. On the baseball field, in between pitches, Roy slurped away. At recess he'd try to worm his way in with a bunch of us boys, mostly listening to us talk, everyone else being cool, keeping their hands in their pockets—except Fingers.

Fingers just kept, well, being Fingers, until that day when Bruzzy Fleck did something good by being bad.

In the lunchroom Fingers was at the end of the table, sucking and twirling away as usual between bites. Nobody was giving him much attention. What could you say? "Fingers taste good today, Fingers?" Bruzzy came out of the line and went to the next table to eat. As he put down his tray, he looked over towards us and saw Fingers. Soon Bruzzy got that nasty look; his pupils, as they usually did when he planned to do something bad, started to jump around in his eyes, bobbing up and down like people doing the wave at a football game. He gave us one of his patented "watch this" signs that also warned, "Don't you dare let on you know what I'm going to do."

Slowly, quietly—and this was hard for a big bozo like Bruzzy—he crept up behind Fingers. Now he was standing right behind him.

Bruzzy waited for Fingers to finish a bite and put his fingers back in position. Then, when they were all the way in his mouth, he suddenly grabbed Fingers' head in his two hands, the left hand pressing down hard from the top, the right hand pushing up from the bottom, underneath the chin. Fingers let out a scream, the loudest, most pain-filled scream I had ever heard. Bruzzy had forced him to bite down so hard on his two fingers that when he took them out of his mouth everyone started shouting, "He bit off his fingers! He bit off his fingers!" "Gross!" "Right through the bone!"

Someone called the school nurse. Fingers lay on the bench, crying and screaming, endlessly repeating, "My fingers! My fingers!"

Of course, he hadn't bitten off his fingers, though it looked like he had come close. But from that day on Fingers never sucked his fingers anymore. Oh, he would start to, but then his eyes would begin to twitch, his hands shake, and he'd look right and left, as if expecting Bruzzy Fleck to be standing behind him, ready to crunch his head down. Just the thought of it was enough to stop Fingers from sucking and twirling.

He never sucked his fingers again. Bruzzy had *cured* him. Bruzzy Fleck! The bully! Two days before school stopped for the summer, Norma Roth suggested that we stop calling Fingers "Fingers." So, for two wonderful days in school that year, he was called Roy. As for Bruzzy, he kept on being bad. Still, in one wonderful second, just like Fingers'—I mean Roy's—two wonderful days, Bruzzy had proved that a coin has two sides.

Chapter 10

Feeling Better

"We know about how something good comes out of something bad," the kids said as I entered Charlie's Corner with my wife Norma, who often joined me for the story telling.

"We're feeling better this week."

"Yeah, but this new treatment still sucks!"

"But what are ya gonna do?"

"That needle they use is—" and with this Freddie measured out a rough three inches with his thumb and index finger.

Not to be outdone, Veronica, Amanda's newfound friend, raised the stakes to a foot. And within minutes, with the boys joining in, the needle had grown exponentially until it was longer than a baseball bat.

"And ya know where they put it?" With this, the unholy trinity of Tommy, Grant, and Freddie stuck out their backsides. Now, whether that was the actual destination of the needle I did not know. I'd have to ask Dr. Graham-Pole about it. By now everyone, including one of the nurses whom I had secretly nicknamed "Ms. Stern," was convulsed with

laughter. Edgar's line from Shakespeare's King Lear *came to my head—"The worst returns to laughter."*

When a surface calm had been restored, Amanda, picking up on the remarks that had greeted me when Norma and I arrived, said, "So, since we're all feeling better, how 'bout an adventure story?"

"Have I ever told you about the snakes in Arkansas, with the country girls and the old fogey school teacher?"

"No," then "Please," Norma and the kids sang in unison.

⟿

Going West

In January 1954, the Bell Telephone Workers of Philadelphia went on strike for higher wages, and now, with Dad's first pay raise in years, my mother had decided we could splurge, and so for the summer of 1954 we did not vacation in Wildwood. The Porettas, whose cottage we always rented, were sorely disappointed. This year we would be going west.

Outside the car, the United States passed by. Inside the Dodge we established a hermetically sealed environment A model of dogged consistency as he kept the speedometer at 35, that speed set by divine decree above and which to exceed even by a mile per hour was to court tragedy, Dad gazed intently at the road. Face glued to a map, Mother converted the brave new world ebbing by our window into the abstract, sterile lines and circles of Rand McNally. In the back seat, transformed into a cave by the slits that passed as rear windows in the old car, John and I chatted quietly about those things hidden from parents, the boyhood secrets and ambitions that alone give a sense of uniqueness, of imaginary power to the powerless, to minors longing to be adults, longing to drive the Dodge themselves, to rev it to 50, to force other cars off the road and impress a line of girls along the side.

Six days later we arrived in Tulsa, Oklahoma, where, our host told us, everyone was at least "one-eighth Indian" and proud of it; Tulsa, whose front and backyards hosted oil wells; Tulsa, Oklahoma, the West, outside those four blocks in Philly.

Billy Taylor, a jolly man, his face in a continual smile, a widower for twenty years, was glad to have us. Now retired, he was the perfect host, devoting every waking second to us. When we got up the next morning, by our bed stand was a schedule for each day of our stay. Tuesday promised: "8 AM—country-fried breakfast / 10–12 noon—tour of Oklahoma Indian Museum / noon–1:30—lunch at the El Grando Restaurant / 1:30–4:00— visit to cattle ranch"—a list of events right up until bedtime. We were especially drawn to an entry for day three of our stay: "9 AM–6 PM—boys go to Aunt Minn's in the hills and meet local girls." Any request for an explanation—just what did "meet local girls" mean?—was met with howls of generous laughter from Billy. We awaited Thursday with much anticipation, if not with a little fear. Local girls?

On Thursday, Billy took us to the bus station: John and I were to travel by ourselves to Aunt Minn's, an old family friend who lived in a small town in the hills just north of the border between Oklahoma and Arkansas. On the way, we had a good chance to speculate about what Aunt Minn's would be like, about those local girls, and also just to enjoy the freedom of traveling by ourselves from the Oklahoma flatlands and then up sharply graded roads, right into the heart of what we had heard was hillbilly country. At any moment we expected to see moonshiners and their stills. What we saw, instead, was a jarring contrast between the magnificent scenery—the rolling hills, the valleys laden with trees, swift-moving mountain streams cutting beneath the road and roaring out the opposite side—and rundown homes, front yards littered with rotting cars and abandoned refrigerators, outhouses, sullen people who barely looked up as the bus rolled by.

Aunt Minn met us at the bus stop. Nothing sullen about her. On the drive to her house, we found out that she had been a schoolteacher all her life, retiring here to the hills for peace and quiet. Ten years ago, however, she had come out of her retirement and was now the sole teacher in the district's one-room schoolhouse, her class of twenty ranging from first grade to high school. She was a thin woman, but not frail. She must have been near eighty, yet her walk was lively. She gave you all her attention, devouring everything you said, even the most mundane answers to her questions. She was all questions, questions upon questions, the "Socrates of the hills" as she billed herself.

Nestled in a thick grove of trees, with a mountain stream literally dividing the front yard in two, Minn's house was as neat as a pin. It shone. Everything had its place. Here, in this hillbilly land, was someone whose living room was lined with books on three sides; only a large fireplace on the back wall prevented her library from encircling the entire room. On the dining table, by the kitchen sink, resting precariously on the rim of the tub in the bathroom, everywhere you looked, were books with markers saving her place.

During lunch we learned that Aunt Minn's interests were wide. At present, she was reading four books—the history of British rule in India, folk medicine of the Ozarks, the poetry of Emily Dickinson, and a biography of Henry Ford. Just as we were about to clear the table, she pointed out the window where the wind was now starting to blow through the mountain ash. "You know, boys, out there's the greatest book of them all. You can take that from an old lady."

"Now it's time to meet the girls," she finally announced, beckoning us to follow her out the door. A half mile down the dirt road we came to one of those hillbilly shacks, and there, sitting on the front porch, dressed in their Sunday best, were two large teenage girls. Large girls with broad shoulders, thick necks and arms, they looked like they could wallop us in wrestling. Very large girls who, the moment they spotted us, came leaping from the porch, hands outstretched, saying "Howdy!" in unison—just the way we imagined, way back in the city, people from the hills of Arkansas greeted each other.

"I'm Alice—you boys like horses?"

"I'm Betty—I'm asking the same as my sister."

As this point in my life I hadn't much to do with girls. John even less. On top of it, the only horse John and I had ever rode was Bruce VanZant's, the one his father used to plow the acre next to their house.

"Sure, we like horses. I'm John and this is my brother Sid."

Aunt Minn said good-bye and reminded us that dinner would be at five.

Before we could say a word, Alice grabbed my hand and ran towards the small barn behind their house. Betty followed with John right behind her. In the barn stood what looked like four ponies, little horses, "mountain steeds" as Alice called them.

"Where's the saddle," I said, trying to sound experienced.

The girls laughed. "We don't use no saddle." The girls mounted their horses bareback. Then, they had to dismount and help John and me get on. Once on, though, we felt fine since the horses were standing still.

But when Betty and Alice shouted, "Yip," all four horses sped out, running two abreast across the yard. Bouncing up and down, John and I barely hung on. John was green; I was too. The sight of us clinging to the horses, every few minutes slipping off and then pulling ourselves back up, drove Alice and Betty into gales of laughter. Even the ponies were enjoying it, for they seemed to relish each new lurch as the trail twisted and turned.

"Whoa!" A command from the girls brought all four horses to a halt. In front of us flowed a slow-moving river. Before we knew it, the girls had dismounted and taken off their dresses right in front of us. They were wearing swimsuits underneath.

"Come in, guys!" Betty shouted.

"Strip!" Alice commanded, laughing.

"Strip?" John and I mouthed silently to each other.

"Come on, the water won't wait all day."

John explained, "I think she means take our shirts and shoes off." So strip we did, with the girls once again pulling us by the hand as we approached the bank.

"Is it cold?" This struck them as terribly funny. That traitor John laughed.

We were about to jump in when John shrieked, "What's that?" There, at the edge of the river the waters were roiling. Peering closer, we saw dozens of snakes feeding in the shallow inlets carved in the riverbank.

"Snakes!" I screamed. The girls remained unruffled.

"Oh, there's always moccasins there," Alice answered, as if this were the most normal thing, as if, somehow, a stream would be incomplete without moccasins.

"Moccasins?"

"Yes, silly, moccasins. You ain't afraid of them, are you?

I didn't wait for John. "You bet I'm afraid."

Like a mother reassuring a child, Alice announced, "Well, you needn't be. Them moccasins always stay right at the bank. We just jump over 'em and swim down the center of the river."

Further reassurance came from her sister. "They won't go out there. The water's too fast and cold."

In a second both girls had leaped from the bank and were swimming down the middle of the river, the area off-limits to the snakes, waving for us to follow. Maybe these girls, born in these backwoods, knew what they were talking about. Holding hands, John and I dove past the snakes, clearing them by a veritable mile, leaving them content to feed on helpless bugs cowardly cleaving to the bank's still shores.

We had taken three trips so far—in the car to Tulsa, on the bus to Arkansas, and that wild pony ride. Going down that river was the best. You could swim or flow with the current. The banks and the forests passed by, and, at a more stately pace, the hills followed. We swam in pairs, then changed formation and made our way in a single line. Changing once more, we created a phalanx of four braving the river's modest flow. When the current slowed, or the river emptied into temporary ponds, we floated leisurely on our backs, talking about school, about friends, about "back there" as the girls called Philadelphia, about all those silly and wonderful things young people share. We dunked each other; John and I pretended to be snakes and attacked the girls' feet with tickles. Then it was off again into the current.

Now the river became broad, and Alice explained that a half-mile ahead was a dam. The steady flow gave us just enough of a push to make swimming almost effortless.

"What's that?" I asked Betty, noticing what looked like a long stick floating ten feet or so behind us. Before she had a chance to reply, John shouted out, "It's a moccasin!"

"Naw, they always stay near the bank," Betty assured him without looking back.

"It's a moccasin, I tell you!" I'm sure it was, perhaps a cold-fancying, fast-moving water moccasin, an iconoclast defying custom—but a moccasin, nevertheless. Without ever turning back again, all four of us were off, racing for the dam, not wanting to trust the faster exit by the banks. For all we knew, the moccasin's brothers and sisters might be waiting there. For all we knew, it was still there behind us. Probably gaining speed. There, behind us, deciding which of us to bite first. Country and city distinctions broke down. Arkansas and "back there" were indistinguishable. Locals and visitors—who cared? We were four terrified kids desperate to reach the dam and salvation.

Now the dam was just ahead. The mixture of fear, cold water, and swimming at full speed had had its effect. Cramps set in. Betty's right leg was numb, as was John's left arm. I felt like my whole body had fallen asleep, and Alice could barely propel herself through the water. The snake must be gaining on us. At last we saw the dam. Chests heaving, legs cramping, we breathlessly pulled ourselves onto its side, free at last from the dangerous waters alive with untold moccasins.

We invited Betty and Alice to join us for dinner. After Aunt Minn called Billy Taylor to ask if we could spend the night, I took her aside.

"Could Emily and Betty stay a bit?"

"That would be natural," she observed, and then added, "Would you like to hear some poetry?"

Sitting on the hearth, she read from that copy of Emily Dickinson I had seen earlier in the day. The poems memorized, sometimes she looked at us directly, the way a speaker eyes an audience. At other times she retreated into herself, focused on the book in her hands, the portrait of an old woman who, like the long-dead poet, had surely known love and isolation in her day. Emily Dickinson of Amherst, Massachusetts, lived again here in the hills of southern Arkansas.

John stretched out on the floor, serene in a way I had never seen before. Betty sat nearby, her head resting on her knees, lost in thought. I felt Alice put her hand in mine.

The nurses arrived to bring the children to their beds.

"I'm gonna dream of those Arkansas hills tonight."

"Me too. And floating down that river, without the snakes, of course."

"I'm gonna jump right over the snakes. They'll be snapping at me but I'll be sailing right over their heads."

"Yeah, into that cool water."

"Mrs. Homan, did you know your husband had a girl-friend, that girl who held his hand after the poetry?"

"I bet they did more than hold hands!"

"I took a trip like that once."

As these and other comments faded down the hall, Norma and I sat alone in Charlie's Corner. I felt her hand in mine, just as forty years ago Alice had held my hand as we sat listening to Aunt Minn reading Emily Dickinson's poems.

"You know, Sid, that was a great story you told the kids."

"I meant it for you, too."

"Tell me one on the way home."

"You want a story?"

"Yeah."

"Let me think." A pause. "I've got one. Let me tell you the story about **Staying with Aunt Grace**."

⚜

Mother tried to hide the fact that she came from a Polish family who lived in Tamacqua, Pennsylvania, in the heart of the anthracite coal-mining district. When she moved to Philadelphia, she left behind her sister, our Aunt Grace. Aunt Grace never married, although she tried everything she could to attract a husband. She dyed her hair; one visit it would be blonde, the next red. The medicine cabinet in her bathroom was filled with bottle upon bottle of nail polish, nail-polish remover, hair coloring, face powder, rouge, cleansing creams, along with packs of eyeliners and tubes of lipstick.

"Aunt Grace could stock a store out of that cabinet," John said.

"She's got so much in there you can smell the stuff when you drive up," I replied, trying to top him.

Aunt Grace's house was halfway up a steep street, where all the buildings came right up to the sidewalk, one of those upstate houses, with long, narrow rectangular windows, fake brick siding, and a high-gabled roof. Six steps led to the front door; in the back was a fenced-in garden, with a gate at the far end. Beyond the gate lay the scarred land where coal had been strip-mined, a treeless landscape dotted with steep pits, some of them 100 yards across, filled with water that had turned brackish-red or copper-green, even yellow. Local people, who owed their living to the mines, called the area ugly. John and I found it terrifying, like an alien planet, yet in a way compelling.

Beyond the gate rose the Allegheny Mountains, with those abandoned coal miners' caves John and I were forbidden to enter.

On the first floor of Aunt Grace's house was a sitting room; a very small, never-used dining room; and a long, large kitchen, in the center of which was a wood-burning stove that also heated the house. On the second floor were two bedrooms, along with the bathroom and that famous cabinet bursting with cosmetics. Above, on the third floor, was the attic, where John and I slept—a wonderful place that with its high roof looked like a tent. At the top of the roof was a glass window through which you could see the sky. The rumor was that Aunt Grace's former boyfriend—her *only* boyfriend probably—had installed it for her.

Grace was a collector—of everything. She was the one who got John and me started with bottle caps. Hers was the master collection, over two hundred caps, each one different, some going back to the 1920s when she was in high school. Matchbooks, dolls, bottle openers, stamps, coins, movie posters, miniature books, doll houses, doll furniture, postcards, porcelain figures, candles, teacups, license plates, shoes, gloves, jack-in-the-boxes, children's toys, fortunes from fortune cookies from every meal she had ever had in a Chinese restaurant—she collected everything!

A thin, bony woman, with skin that stretched tight on her face, she smelled of powder and perfume; her cheeks were so red you would swear she was wearing a mask. She looked unnatural, like a middle-aged doll. Totally self-absorbed, her only topics of conversation were the goings-on among her neighbors whom we did not know, the price of this or that at the grocery store at the bottom of the hill, who was working and who had been laid off in the coal mines. She was also expert in the latest fads in facial creams or toenail polishes. And food—the meal she had just cooked or the next one she planned for dinner. If you mentioned something about yourself, an event or place in the "big city"—every place outside her coal-mining town was dismissed as the "big city"—if you referred to anything existing beyond Tamacqua, she either found something in her small world that was like it or better. After a cursory nod that seemed to say, "I heard what you said—there, I've done my part," she would steer the conversation back to something that interested her. In doing so, Aunt Grace was not so much annoying as comic, unconsciously and pathetically so.

Visits to Aunt Grace's were always the same. As we drove towards her house, there would be a silent rustle of lace curtains in the neighbors' windows; you'd see clearly the hand that had parted them and, less clearly, a dim face now framed by the opening, peering out at you. As Dad drove down the street at his usual agonizingly slow speed, those parting curtains produced something of a falling domino effect, opening and closing.

We settled quickly into Aunt Grace's routine. Three meals anchored the day. The kitchen stove was the physical and spiritual center of her universe. Life in Tamacqua was boring. From the sitting room you could watch the goings-on in the street outside. Around the stove, you listened to Aunt Grace go on and on in painstaking detail about Tamacqua. Daily trips to the grocery store, always in the middle of the afternoon. A visit to the Chinese restaurant the final night came none too soon. The sisters argued over who would pay the bill, and, of course, Aunt Grace saved all of the fortunes from the cookies. After dinner, we gathered around the television set—a luxury in those days—and watched *Milton Berle, Arthur Godfrey,* or *The Goldbergs.* Mornings we cleaned the house. Aunt Grace's habit was to give us "assignment sheets" with very specific duties, such as "take out drawers and dust inside the bureau," or "clean light bulbs in bathroom" or "sweep behind all second-floor doors." Dad was "allowed out" after lunch. He would walk the streets of Tamacqua, striking up conversations with perfect strangers, attracting attention by the odd way he smoked his pipe.

Dad always smoked his pipe on his after-dinner walk through our neighborhood since mother wouldn't allow "that thing" indoors. During World War II my mother was appointed warden of the four blocks that formed our neighborhood, her job being to sound the alert if German bombers flew over the city. She saw to it that when we had a night air-raid drill, everyone turned off all their house lights. The rationale was that a dark city presented the most difficult target for Hitler's air force. Dad was a creature of habit, and one night, just as he was about to leave the house, an air-raid alarm sounded.

"Where do you think you're going?" Mother bellowed at him.

"You know, May Elaine, I always take a walk after dinner."

"Right now? Smoking that thing?"

"You know I always smoke my pipe."

"And what if a German pilot should see it lit? Everyone else's lights are off, and there you go, waltzing right out the door, pipe lit, burning away, giving those Nazis a perfect target."

"Oh, come on—"

"Just our luck they're going to attack tonight, and here you are, the perfect target."

Dad looked helplessly at John and me. Mom stood blocking the door, hands on her hips. Then, we saw a smile gather on Dad's face. He put out the pipe. Mother flushed a smile a triumph. Too soon, for the next instant Dad pushed the tobacco a little tighter in the bowl and relit the pipe. Mother was fuming.

"And just what do you think you're doing?"

Dad looked at us with a "you'll see." Very calmly, clearly enjoying every second, he turned the pipe upside down. It continued burning yet there was no red glow. As he sauntered out the door we knew that tonight we would be safe; tonight the Germans would not bomb Philadelphia. Dad sailed through the crisp night air, puffing away, the smoke curling up and around the pipe, the embers in the bowl invisible to the enemy. From that day on, long after Germany had surrendered, Dad continued to smoke his pipe turned downward. Now he sailed through the streets of Tamacqua, acknowledging the residents' stares, the puzzled expressions, and savoring his rare victory over Mother ten years ago.

If pipe smoking brought Dad freedom from Aunt Grace's regime, John and I found relief each afternoon during the hour before dinner when we were allowed to explore the strip-mined land—we called it "the moonscape"—beyond her backyard, reminded, as always, not to go beyond the foothills, the gateway to the mountains and those forbidden abandoned miners' caves. That sterile, treeless world, the ground rutted from the trucks that had long ago abandoned the place, showed no signs of life, no sounds, only deep pits, the last bastion of the strip mines, their depth a measure of the coal company's determination that going any deeper would not be "cost-effective."

Ahead of us loomed the Allegheny Mountains, thick with trees, green in summer and brilliant in fall with the hues of the mountain ash, the only defect the bare swath, from our perspective no wider than a pencil, running from the base to the top to accommodate power lines. Every dark spot among the trees signified a former miner's cave, and on this issue John and I were in dispute—he counted six, I seven.

In our imaginations the moonscape between Aunt Grace's garden gate and those green mountains became a paradise. Waterless pits metamorphosed to staging areas for hide-and-seek; we skimmed stones on the surfaces of pits transformed to lakes. Clumps of dirt became hand grenades in mock wars. Best of all, digging even a half-foot into the soil exposed all sorts of treasures abandoned by the miners: a still-operable cigarette lighter, a copy of *The Policeman's Gazette* with pictures of almost naked women, coins, tools, a watch, a bronze belt-buckle carved like the star of Texas, a pouch of chewing tobacco, hundreds of empty cigarette packages that for us quickly formed a collection rivaling our bottle caps, a photograph of a family of twelve posing beside a large black Nash, numerous pocket knives.

Against all odds, small crocuses pushed their way through the rocks, and in the late summer weeds, growing like a field of wheat, caught the strong winds blowing from the mountains. Once we stole some vegetable seeds from Aunt Grace, tools, ten buckets of dirt, and a bag of fertilizer we found unopened in a small shed, and planted a garden near the foothills in a culvert formed by a dried-up stream. Hidden from the world, certainly hidden from Aunt Grace, that garden gave us an excuse to venture into the forbidden mountains to get water from a stream that poured down from the top before it went underground near the base.

On one of those trips for water we discovered a cave halfway up the mountain. Shining a flashlight into the dark, we could see that the corridor ran two hundred feet or so straight inside and then went in three directions. We dared each other to step inside. It wasn't Aunt Grace's rule inhibiting us, but rather our own sense of unease. Unnatural, an intrusion dug years ago into the mountain when the mines were in full operation, the deserted shaft now seemed positively evil—an abomination. Yet it also lured us.

"My God, it's six," I said. We raced back to Aunt Grace's. To be even one minute late would violate her schedule. John and I were now halfway there, at the very midpoint of the moonscape. Ahead was the freshly painted white fence, the garden with its three perfect rows, and inside Mother, Dad, and Aunt

Grace around the kitchen stove waiting for us. Behind us were the mountains, the Alleghenies, the first barrier to settlers moving west, now lit in garish hues by the sun making its last stand. Somewhere in that imperceptible distance lay the cave.

"Look!" John cried.

"Where?"

"There," he said pointing in the cave's direction. A light was flashing, no bigger than a pinprick, but clearly flashing. At us! With a message?

"Come on, John—we've got no time for that now."

Aunt Grace clicked her teeth ominously. "I don't know what you boys see in that godforsaken place." Apologies made for being late, we settled into the evening dinner. Aunt Grace allowed for no after-dinner conversation. The moment the final bite was taken everyone rose and fell to their assigned tasks of clearing, sweeping, washing, drying, and stacking. Back in the sitting room playing canasta, we kept one eye on the cards and the other on the neighbors who, behind their own lace curtains, were probably playing canasta too, with one eye on us. At eight, Dad was released for his upside-down pipe-smoking voyage along the streets of Tamacqua. As he posed in the door to say goodnight, he lit that pipe the same way, and with the same savor of success, he had done that night when Hitler's Luftwaffe was threatening the city. Mother pretended not to notice.

"Can we go out?" I asked.

"And what would you do?" Aunt Grace asked, surprised, shocked that anyone, at this time of day, would want to venture into the outside world.

"We'll stay in the backyard."

"Yeah, getting a bit of fresh air after that fine meal of yours, Aunt Grace," John added with a nice touch.

Once outside, we tried to spot the light we had seen from the cave, but the mountains remained dark and silent.

Suddenly John said, "Wonder what it would be like to go into that cave at night?"

Even though I had had the same thought, I gave him an expression that said, "Now, why would you think of such a stupid thing?" Inside we could see Mother and Aunt Grace sitting by the stove, drinking tea, talking just as they must have when they were young years ago.

"How can Aunt Grace live in a place like this and not want to go exploring?" John asked.

"Beats me," I said, half pushing him as I moved towards the kitchen door. Just before entering the house, we both turned around and looked back towards the cave. No flashing light.

An hour later, before we headed to bed, Aunt Grace gave us each a hot brick that had been heated on the stove and then wrapped in a thick towel. "To keep you comfy," she said cheerfully as we kissed her goodnight.

There was no heat in the attic but the hot brick under your sheets at the foot of the bed kept everything nice and warm until you fell asleep. John and I lay on our backs, staring at the moon shining through the window. Below, we could hear Dad come in and join the sisters in the kitchen. In a few moments, all three were laughing. John and I just lay there, without talking. When the wind outside picked up, the old house began to groan. Now the bricks had cooled so that we could rest our toes on them and feel the heat making its way through the towel. Through the skylight we could see wisps of black clouds blowing across the moon. Dad and Mother started upstairs, while Aunt Grace stayed behind in the kitchen, putting the finishing touches on her day. We heard our parents' door shut and, later, Aunt Grace go into her bedroom. The sky had cleared and five stars circled the moon. The wind was even stronger now, and there was a tapping sound on the roof—probably a tree branch caught on the shingles. John had fallen asleep, or so I thought, and in a minute or so I followed suit.

Suddenly, he was shaking me with, "Let's sneak outside."

"What?"

"Come on. I couldn't get to sleep. I was just faking. So, now you're up too, let's sneak outside."

Minutes later we were dressed. We could hear Aunt Grace snoring. In the kitchen a homey red glow came from the stove. There was a flashlight by the back door.

"The caves?"

"Yeah, the caves."

"We'll never get another chance."

The town was asleep; lace curtains hung limp in their windows. A crisp wind from the mountains blew across the moonscape, which now seemed more unreal than ever. The only sound came from bits of coal crunching beneath our shoes. Without speaking, we moved toward the mountains. We knew tonight we would challenge, *disobey*, Aunt Grace's most sacred rule—we would go into the cave! In that foolish, suicidal way of young people, we rejoiced.

Now far away, our maiden Aunt Grace lay snoring in her bed, face still caked with rouge, eyebrows teased and blackened, lips painted a garish red, hair doused with her favorite rose water. Aunt Grace, sound in her bed, never suspecting, but dreaming of the carpenter, now long dead, who once had romanced her, giving false promise of marriage before leaving, his parting gift that wondrous window in the attic. How many nights, when she was alone in that house, after we had departed, had Aunt Grace lain in that attic bed, her body warmed by a hot brick? How often had she looked through that window and thought of the carpenter, dreaming of her cavalier as the moon passed overhead? Sleep tight, be comfy, Aunt Grace, for tonight John and I are going to the cave, toward our destiny.

"I bet there are a million passageways inside," John observed as we pointed the flashlight into the entrance.

"Billions."

"What if we get lost?"

With the smugness of an older brother, I cut him off with, "I've thought of that," as I produced a piece of chalk from my pocket.

"Chalk?"

"Yeah, chalk, " I replied with mock anger as if he should have been able to figure out how a single piece of chalk would keep us from getting lost. My inspiration had come from a comic-book story in which the hero, on a mission to rescue a boy lost in a labyrinth, retraced his path by following in reverse order the numbers he had written on the walls. John agreed it was a great idea.

Once inside the cave we walked the two hundred or so feet to where the path divided into three tunnels.

"Let's take the one to the left," John ventured. I dutifully wrote a large "1" five feet down the passageway. There were lots of choices as we moved deeper, and we took turns deciding whether to go right or left, all the time secure in the knowledge that the numbers entered every twenty feet or so would serve for our exit. By number "25" the cave felt colder, damper. Somewhere, hundreds of feet, maybe thousands of feet behind, reached by a random combination of right and left turns, but now in reverse order, was number "1." It was thrilling, dangerous, illegal. If the moonscape was our old world, here was a very different one, a brave new world carved by miners, pioneers we knew only from their abandoned artifacts. The silence was profound. We felt nurtured by the darkness, at one with the dampness.

"Do you suppose if we keep on we'll end up on the other side of the earth?" John asked.

"Without a doubt," I replied, laughing yet also wishing somehow it were true.

When we got to "100," we agreed that enough was enough. Trying to protect our separate egos by letting the other be the first one to say that we should turn back, we spoke almost precisely at the same time.

"Let's go."

After all, this dark place offered only a fraudulent, transitory pleasure. Reality was Aunt Grace's kitchen stove, that building housing the unmarried and the married sister, and that gentle, dear man whom we loved more than anything in the world.

We started tracing the numbers backward, the system working like a charm. We passed "90" and then "80" and "70."

"What if the flashlight fails, Sid? You ever think of that?"

"I saw Aunt Grace put new batteries in the second day we were here." No, the flashlight did not fail.

Instead, it was the numbers that failed, for while we could find "42," there was no "41" or "40," or "39" for that matter. All the numbers before "42" had vanished!

There, at "42" we stopped, *were* stopped, and now, as our fears mounted, we speculated wildly, with little hope any answer would prove true. Was there some malignant force that had taken its revenge on us for disobeying our aunt? The flashlight couldn't last forever. We could try alternate routes, but what if that only led to our getting further lost? As if we could be any more lost than at present?

"Let's use a new number system when we try out the possibilities," I suggested, "so that if one route doesn't lead us to the old numbers, at least we can find our way back to this place."

The moment we wrote the first number on the wall, we realized what had gone wrong. The cave wall was too moist, and instead of drawing clear lines, the chalk dissolved into the rock.

"At least we know it wasn't some evil spirit," I said in a pathetic effort to ease our fear. We started to panic. There was no need to put that panic into words; like twins, John and I knew what the other was thinking, feeling. We both had the same vision: two boys, buried forever hundreds of feet below the surface, starving to death in this abnormal tomb, their cries unheard, our panic changing to desperation and desperation lapsing into madness.

We sat there, stupidly, without a plan. I was barely able to restrain the urge to leap up and start racing insanely around the passageways, foolishly imagining that if we tried enough combinations, somehow chance itself would let us hit on the right one. In fact, I was about to do just that, and John must have sensed it.

"Wait, Sid, I know what to do. Just follow me." I demanded my brother explain; he refused. He was, in effect, ordering me, the older brother, the *favored* son, to agree without any explanation. Grabbing the flashlight, with me following on his heels, John began walking, taking a right turn here, two left turns there, then a right, then a left, then two rights. He moved boldly, indeed, cheerfully, like someone out for a Sunday stroll through a neighborhood he had known all of his life. When I protested, asking if he knew what he was doing, he simply smiled back at me, as if my concern were irrelevant. For all intents and purposes, *he* was now the older brother.

In a few minutes we saw the moonlight at the entrance of the cave. We were free! We hurried back to Aunt Grace's house, joyful, drunk in our salvation, "shush"ing each other as we made our way to the attic. Aunt Grace was still snoring and dreaming. Still warmed by the brick, the bed felt reassuring.

There was no need to talk about what might have happened in the cave—*nothing* had happened. As we were drifting off to sleep, I asked John the inevitable question. "How did you know which path to follow out of the cave?"

"I had no idea what I was doing, Sid—no idea in the world."

Saturday was our final day—day six—with Aunt Grace. Late in the morning, John took a pellet gun he had bought at the store down the street and practiced with it, hitting targets on the moonscape, until lunch.

He had the gun with him when we visited our secret world for the last time. To our delight we saw the light blinking from the cave a half-mile away, beckoning us. We had mastered the cave, so this time we were content to remain in the moonscape without investigating. John cocked the pellet gun to his shoulder.

"Watch this." Aiming carefully, he took a shot. A second later we heard the sound of the pellet striking something metallic. In that same moment the mysterious light went out. We made our way towards the mountains, past the variously colored pits now catching the sun's last rays. There, a hundred feet from the cave, we found a tin can that had been shattered by John's shot.

"Nothing mysterious after all."

CHAPTER II

Reality Returns

Spring break was over, reality returned, and I was eager to see my kids in the Bone Marrow Unit. On my way to Charlie's Corner, John Graham-Pole stopped with bad news. "I wanted to tell you that Tommy won't be there today."

"Why? Anything happen?"

"He's had a seizure and we've put him in Intensive Care."

Entering the room heavyhearted, I was immediately assaulted by the four teenagers, and five new kids. The former raced up to me, pressing close to my face the way young people do when they talk, with "Great to see you again" and "We missed you." Amanda had her head shaven, which she proudly displayed for me, as if this were her badge of admission to the club.

Then James with a sober face said, "They wheeled Tommy out of his room while he was still in his bed."

"I know."

"You know what that means?"

I could manage only a sober "yes."

There were not enough chairs for everyone, and so James, ever the diplomat, suggested that we sit on the floor, on that gaudy rug with the fake Indian design. Those who had to stay in wheelchairs pretended they were sitting. Soon, with the rug as a meager stage set, their imaginations were aglow.

"It's like we're around a campfire at night."

"I'm roasting marshmallows. Want one?" James asked as he pushed an imaginary marshmallow on a stick in my direction.

"Camp food sucks!" one exclaimed, and soon they were swapping horror stories about bad meals, the items of which sounded suspiciously like the hospital fare.

Grant concocted a bizarre tale about Edna, Amanda's friend, falling out of the rowboat and discovering the Lost Atlantis at the bottom of the lake. Someone spread the rumor that Amanda was seen making out with James behind a bush, and Amanda protested as if the rumor encased with the fictive world of the camp were gospel truth. In the darkness surrounding the small circle of the fire two beady eyes were spotted and within minutes Evans had painted a graphic portrait of the monster.

"How about a spooky story? The type they tell at camp."

A spooky story it would be. "Did I ever tell you about **A Fish in the Moonlight***?"*

"A Fish in the Moonlight? That sounds odd," said James, who was now sitting very close to Amanda.

⌘

Things began to change in junior high school. Our voices started to crack, a sure sign that they were moving down to some lower, more "manly" register. The former smooth curve of the neck, not much unlike a girl's, was now interrupted with a bump that, as nature took its course, became the highly prized Adam's apple. When the first few black hairs on the chin or along the cheeks took the place of the peach fuzz that had seen us through elementary school, then manhood was in full flower.

"Hey, Neil, I'll be shaving soon."

"Sid, you shaving?"

"Yeah, got four hairs on my chin—look!"

"Four?"

"Yeah, four."

"Hell, I've had six for two weeks now!'

With that I slunk off, manhood defeated, until that prize-winning six was mine too.

More than a matter of new-grown beards, in junior high boundaries began to move. Not far away—but away, nevertheless. Our four blocks—Roseland Avenue, Fox Chase Pike, Kirkland Street, and Seminole Avenue—relieved only by a trip to Lorimer Park or shopping at the A&P in Jenkintown, expanded. Donald Asher was a new friend in a neighborhood next to ours, whereas before I had only known the Polling family. Donald's mother had a curious speech defect: When she talked it seemed as if her voice was coming out of her nose. There wasn't any Mr. Asher; years ago he had run off with some blonde girl half his age.

John and I also discovered Eli and Yanif Erbing, sons of the caretaker of Lawnview Cemetery. An iron fence with vertical bars just wide enough for young boys to squeeze through surrounded Lawnview. Eli and Yanif showed us a great game involving gravediggers. Now those gravediggers were rough, mean-spirited men, unshaven and always drunk. The game was to taunt them as they dug graves. Angered, they would charge, cursing and swinging their shovels. We would rush to the fence, put one shoulder in the space between the iron bars, waiting in that position until the gravedigger was only a few feet away, and as he lunged, threatening to crack our heads with his shovel, we'd slip through the fence. If you waited until the very last moment—and that took a lot of guts, believe me!—then only one second after you were safely on the other side the gravedigger would come crashing into the fence, his shovel making sparks as it clanged against the bars. Once a shovel came within an inch of Eli's head, and as the gravedigger bellowed, Eli took a bow, to much applause from Yanif, John, and me. On summer evenings Mrs. Erbing would sell lilacs at the cemetery gate. Inside, we boys would play hide-and-seek among the graves.

Now I got to spend nights at new houses, to sleep in strange beds and eat food cooked by other mothers. Johnnie Botstein's father was a wealthy lawyer. A diabetic, Johnnie felt different from the rest of us kids. Perhaps because of his illness, there was a darkness, a cynicism about him, a morbid wit in his every thought that I found strangely appealing, sophisticated. At Johnnie's house you played chess, with Mozart in the background.

Arson Donadarian was Armenian; his family had a picture of Mount Ararat in the living room. Arson's dad owned twenty-seven dry-cleaning stores around the city, and the gossip was that his employees used to dry their condoms along with the customers' laundry. Once at his New Year's Eve party Arson announced, just minutes before midnight, that he was charging everyone five dollars for refreshments. We all had thought the party was free. As the television showed that globe of lights descending to the roof of the triangular building on Times Square, everyone started to mumble, then curse Arson for being so cheap by tricking us into coming. Sensing the crowd's anger, Arson quickly added, "Hey, if you stay after and help clean up, I'll make it only $2!" That was the final insult. No one celebrated the New Year; there was no kissing or ringing bells. Everyone charged out of the house. I stayed. Arson was in tears.

"What did I do wrong, Sid?"

I lied. "Nothing, Arson . . . nothing." Arson was my best buddy.

Connie Armbruster completed my trinity of new friends. Connie had no father; his mother worked as a greeter at a restaurant in town. Connie had the whitest skin imaginable; he was almost an albino. And Connie was crazy in a nice sort of way. When we went to the movies, he'd always go up into the balcony. Once the show started, he'd take out a roll of toilet paper, a jar of peanut butter, and a knife. Putting some of the peanut butter on a few sheets of the paper, he'd fling the mess over the balcony. When it landed below, usually on some kid, everyone around would think—well, you can just imagine what they would think. At least for a few seconds until they discovered the truth. Meanwhile, Connie let forth with a flood of high-pitched laughter, soon to be imitated around the darkened theatre.

Once, when the newsreel showed a picture of Hitler giving a speech, Connie hurled a huge jackknife at the screen, which promptly cut a gaping hole in the fabric. The manager, the sepulchral-looking Mr. Nelson, turned on the lights at once, mounted the stage, and demanded to know who had done it. We all knew, yet no one said a word.

"If no one tells, then you'll all go home. And I won't refund your money either."

"What about if someone tells?" came a voice came from the balcony.

"If someone tells, then I'll give you all a refund."

Silence. Again the same voice from the balcony. "That's not enough."

Desperate to find the guilty party, Mr. Nelson hemmed and hawed and then came out with, "OK, along with the refund I'll show two cartoons and two Flash Gordon episodes next Saturday."

A seemingly new voice from the balcony, "It was Connie Armbruster."

Mr. Nelson kept his word. After a long talk with Connie's mother, he let him off scot-free. Connie was our hero for a few weeks when we realized he was both those voices from the balcony.

I liked these new friends and the freedom they promised. I liked having to take a bus to school. I especially liked looking at girls' breasts. Richard Fasser, Spitty Grossman, the Rupert brothers, Norma Roth, Jimmy Dooley, Mildred Bosshart, Jimmy Neil, not to mention the Klecto children and Bobby Mickle from Roseland Avenue, even Leslie Doober—all these people started to fade, to be replaced by my new buddies, Johnnie Botstein, Arson Donadarian, and Connie Armbruster. The four of us used to walk the railroad tracks to Lorimer Park, pretending to be soldiers on a parade ground singing "You're in the Army Now" and "Cadence Count" as we marched single file, trying to keep our balance on the rails. It was assumed that if you invited one of us to a birthday party, the other three ought to come too. We were a unit, a team, maybe even a single person disguised as four.

I remember the night we would later call "A Fish in the Moonlight." Connie had stolen some bottles of Schmidt's beer from his mother, and Johnnie suggested we meet at midnight, just outside the country club where his father was a member, then sneak inside to drink the beer by the lake in the center of the golf course. I set my alarm clock for eleven-thirty. I remember passing by my brother's room. The door was open, and there he lay, curled around "Stinky," a mere shell of a dog for it had long since lost its stuffing. John looked so young, a baby, and here I was, off to meet my buddies and drink Schmidt's beer, the same beer the factory workers drank. Five black hairs on your chin, a bottle of cold Schmidt's in your hand—hell, you were almost a man, practically one of those high-school guys who drove cars.

Connie, Arson, and Johnnie were waiting for me at the gate. The place was deserted. The clubhouse and restaurant, approached by a winding, tree-lined drive, stood on a hill. The golf course lay in the center, flanked to the left by the lake—our destination. To avoid being seen from the road, we went to the far side. Soon the four of us were stretched out on the soft grass that grew right up to the edge of the water. As the bottles of still-cold beer were passed about, we gave way to those wonderful, comforting adolescent clichés. "Man, this is the life." "Hey, Arson, don't chug the whole thing—leave a drop for me." "All we need is some girls." "Sure you can hold your beer, man?" The conversation flowed from friends, to girls, to teachers, both favorites and despised, to parents, to little brothers and sisters, to predictions of what high school would be like, all this mixed with various boasts, off-color stories, and confessions, true or false, of how light-headed we were feeling. Within thirty minutes the conversation had degenerated to belches, farts, and those inarticulate cries that signal manhood or mating or—more often—just the inexpressible joy of being young. A full moon above, the soft grass underneath, the country club, dark and deserted, standing impotent on the hill beside us, John clutching Stinky in his bed, my mother asleep, never suspecting—this was the life.

Suddenly, impulsively, Connie tore off his clothes down to his underwear, his "last one in" cut short as he hit the water. In quick order we followed, splashing, dunking. Arson leaped on my back, Johnnie on Connie's. Bare-skinned knights, mounted on uncertain steeds, jousting, the object being not to win, not to vanquish an opponent, but to go crashing to the water, dragging your helpless carrier with you.

In a flash our irresponsible paradise was rudely aborted by lights from an approaching car, the telltale red and blue glow from its roof. The cops! Within seconds Arson, Johnnie, and I were racing around the side of the lake, clutching our clothes, and screaming for Connie who, instead of joining us, lay transfixed by the lake, on his back, his lower half in the water, his torso on the land, gleaming in the moonlight, his body luminous and white against the grass-covered shore. By the time we made it to the opposite side of the lake we saw the two cops standing over Connie, looking down at him, the car's lights blinking ominously in the background, the officers in silhouette, Connie's white face and chest aglow in the moonlight.

"What the hell ya think you're doing?"

The cop's ominous question was met with silence.

"Just who the hell you think *you* are?

At last Connie spoke, a single, nonsensical line, but delivered with an eerie conviction. "I'm a fish, a fish in the moonlight."

"What?" the second cop said incredulously.

"A fish in the moonlight."

Both cops retreated to their car to discuss whatever it is cops discuss in that twilight period between the questioning and the arrest. A fish in the moonlight? Was this a joke? Was he a madman? A poor unfortunate in the clutches of some piscatorial delusion? Could he be serious? Was he mocking their authority? Undergoing some self-inflicted humiliation? While the cops were debating, Connie waved to us on the other side of the lake, and then, leaving his clothes behind, began to creep away from the shore. When he was fifty feet from the cops, he broke into a full run, heading straight towards us, implicating Arson, Johnnie, and me.

"That moron! They'll be after us too!"

In a second the cops began to charge around the lake.

"Hey you, you kid, get back here."

"Make me!"

"Why you little—"

We plunged into the forest on the south side of the country club, the law in frantic pursuit.

"Come on, Connie, come on!"

"I got a pain in my side!"

"Shut up, Johnnie, run!"

"I knew I should've stayed home."

"It was your idea."

Our chests were pounding as if our lungs were trying to break through. When Arson fell behind, Connie pushed him angrily. When Johnnie stumbled, we'd all come to a screaming halt, pick him up, and take off again. Put-downs met any complaint about short breath or exhaustion. Every three or four hundred yards we were confronted with forks in the path. The choice was delegated to Arson. Behind us the cops were cursing loudly, thrashing through bushes that hindered their path but through which we passed with ease. Without shoes, however, Connie began to cry in pain and we were forced to stop. The forest was silent; we assumed the cops had given up.

"I need shoes!" Connie moaned as he hoped up and down on one foot, holding the other in his hand to squeeze out the hurt. "I need shoes, I tell you!"

"Where the hell are we?"

"Damn, Connie's got to get some shoes. Look at him."

"How the hell we gonna find shoes in the forest?"

"At this hour."

In the distance we saw a light, then a small house incongruously fronting the path. Arson knocked and in a few seconds an elderly man appeared in pajamas and a nightcap, like a character from some Grimm fairy tale. His face was grotesque, his nose on an angle, warts rampant on both cheeks, and deep furrows in his brow.

"Bit late boys," he said motioning us in.

I apologized for us and then, pointing to Connie who waited just outside the door, reduced to a pair of underwear, I asked if our strange host had an old pair of shoes we could borrow or perhaps buy.

"Let me see, fellows," he said, retreating to a backroom. When he turned from us, I noticed he had a hump on his back and that the left leg was so much shorter than the right that for balance he was forced to wear a shoe mounted on a platform. For a moment I imagined that this forest was also the home for more oddly-shaped people, exiles living a marginal existence in ancient huts by the path, their boredom and isolation broken only when kids like us, fleeing the law or in search of adventure, passed by. Soon we heard furniture being moved, along with cries of frustration as the old man searched boxes and shelves. Every once in a while he would ask himself, "Shoes, *shoes*, now what did I do with those damn shoes?"

After fifteen minutes or so, he reappeared, a broad smile on his face.

"This'll do ya, just fine," he said, holding out a shoebox.

"How much?" Johnnie asked, afraid to try his luck by assuming the shoes were a gift.

"I reckon a dollar will do it."

Between us we had a dollar in change. We thanked him and once outside tore open the box. Inside were a pair of bright red ballet slippers.

"Ballet slippers!" Connie moaned. "A girl's! And they're red!"

As we turned to protest, the lights went out. In the darkness the little house almost melted into the forest. Let me tell you— it was spooky, as if the house and the old man had never existed.

When Connie put on the slippers, Johnnie let out with, "You look *marvelous* in them, Connie darling," and soon it was all Arson and I could do to keep them from coming to blows. But there was no time for a fight; we heard footsteps coming towards us.

"The cops—not again!" Arson cried plaintively. We were off, Connie leading the way, the streak of his white body dotted at the feet with two red blurs. This time Connie took on Arson's role of choosing between forks in the path. Clouds now covered the moon and we had to feel our way along the path, the bushes our only guide. Run as we would there were always those footsteps behind us.

A half hour later we made two discoveries. We had circled the forest and wound up at the country club lake. And the footsteps turned out to be two shaggy dogs chasing us; once we stopped, they covered us with slobbery greetings. Both had a special fondness for the almost-naked Connie, and we made jokes about their being attracted by those red ballet slippers.

Covered with scratches, exhausted, still we were in a happy mood. There was no sign of the cops, and so, once again, we lay down on the lake's grassy shore.

"You know that feeling you get when you put tinfoil on your back teeth and bite down?"

"Yeah, it hurts like hell."

"Yeah, it hurts—of course, it hurts."

"So?"

"So, when you stop biting down, then you feel good again. In fact, better than you did before. It's like the hurt from the tinfoil almost makes you double glad you're not biting down any more."

"What's the point?"

"Well, like right now. It's almost worth it having been chased by those cops 'cause now we're free—well—it just feels good."

"You mean, you feel free."

"Yeah."

"Why didn't you say that in the first place instead of getting into all this tinfoil crap."

"I was just trying to capture the moment," Johnnie said with a poet-like wave of the hand, imitating Miss Keitel, our English teacher. We had a good laugh at that.

"Were you scared in the forest?'

"Naw."

"The crazy old man?"

"Naw."

"The way his house seemed to vanish?"

"I told you—no!"

"Me neither."

The clouds had scattered and now the sky was covered with stars. For a time we lay there in silence, each in private thought. I imagined Connie was wishing he had a father, or dreaming of that pet snake he kept in his locker at school. Johnnie was hearing Mozart in the back of his head or wandering through the labyrinth in the gardens his father had built for him when he was ten. Arson was thinking of Susie Beard, his girlfriend, whose father wouldn't let him take her out because, we suspected, he didn't want her marrying an Armenian. One of us used to go to the Beard's, pretending to be Susie's date, while Arson waited just down the street. I was wondering how long we would remain friends, or even stay in touch. What a strange quartet we were! Johnnie with diabetes and given to brooding. Arson, someday to be heir to twenty-seven dry cleaning stores. Connie, crazy as a loon, doubtless possessed with an artist's imagination but right now content to be the circus performer juggling before him two well-worn red ballet slippers. And me? If only for now, here with my buddies of the night, a middle-schooler with five black manly hairs on his face, the residue of Schmidt's beer on his breath—*belonging* with boys who had taken an illegal swim. Sidney, who for Friday upon Friday had stayed home, there in the comforting womb of his family, imagining that was all there was in life, all that needed to be. Sidney, who had already adopted his father's habit of shutting the blinds while it was still early twilight, as if to close out the world surrounding 605 Roseland Avenue. Sidney, past midnight, two miles from home, staring at the sky, surrounded by his buddies, indifferent to the consequences.

Once more we were interrupted by the lights of a car approaching the lake.

"No! The cops! Not again!" we cried.

"Wait, I know that car!" I shouted. The ping-ping-ping of the engine was unmistakable. Our 1938 Dodge. No 1950s car could make that sound. Was it Mother or Dad? That was the question.

"Hello, boys."

"Dad?"

"I woke up, went to check on you, and found you gone."

"But how'd you know we were here?

"Yeah, how'd you know, Mr. Homan?" Connie joined in.

"Well, boys, let's just say I figured that this is where I'd go if I were your age."

After dropping off Connie, Arson, and Johnnie, Dad and I drove home in silence. I knew he wasn't angry like Mother would have been. Dad wasn't angry—he understood. I looked over at him. His dark hair spotted with gray. His hands, rough from working with wires and tape, resting gently on the wheel. As always, he drove slowly, steadily; Dad never hurried through life. Every once in a while he'd look over, sometimes smiling at me, sometimes patting my head with an inaudible "Sonny"— I was always "Sonny" to him, never Sid. He began to hum his favorite song from the big-band era, Bunny Berrigan's "I Can't

Get Started." In a few minutes both of us were quietly singing those lyrics I had learned from Dad.

> I've gone around this world in a plane.
> I've seen revolutions in Spain.
> The North Pole I have charted,
> Still I can't get started with you.

As we pulled into the driveway, Dad was imitating Bunny on the trumpet while I crooned:

> I've been consulted by Franklin D.
> Greta Garbo has asked me to tea.
> I've got a house—it's a showplace,
> Still I can't get no place with you.

We sat awhile in the car. As we got out, Dad cautioned me, "Now be real quiet going upstairs. You wouldn't want to wake your mother. She doesn't need to know, Sonny."

Dad understood. I kissed him on the cheek and tiptoed up the stairs. Twelve steps in all. My room was on the right. John's to the left. I could hear Dad downstairs, locking the back door and then, as he always did, jiggling the front-door handle, just to make sure it was locked as well.

⌁

Outside Charlie's Corner we heard the muted voices of
nurses, the loud buzzer sounding from someone's monitor

*coming unplugged, and at the far end of the hall the clatter
of plates as the kitchen staff brought trays of the despised food
to unwilling diners.*

*Calling me by the most popular of my several names in
Charlie's Corner, one of the new kids broke the silence. "That
story was scary, Mr. Sid."*

"Tell us another one."

"Yeah, a funny one this time."

"With your three friends."

"And put in your brother John, too."

I leaped at the chance. "Did I ever tell you a story called
Put That Cigarette Out*?"*

In the 1930s Willow Grove had been a fashionable amusement park where the wealthy people from the city listened to
John Philip Sousa's military band. Twenty years later the park
catered to families, the perfect place to visit on a summer
evening since the thick elm trees kept out the heat of the day.

Once while Connie, Johnnie, Arson, and I were there,
halfway through the evening the three of us became separated
from Arson. Try as we might, we couldn't find him in the
crowd. Connie had a bright idea. He went to the park office,
told them some fishy story about having an emergency and
needing to locate Arson Donadarian right away. In a few minutes we all heard over the loudspeakers, "Ladies and gentlemen,
will an Arson—" There was a pause. Then, "Just a second. This

is a very strange name. *Very* strange. I can't quite say it." Another silence, followed by a "Dona . . . dona . . . dona" as the announcer struggled with the pronunciation. A few more feeble attempts followed by, "This is the craziest name I've ever seen." With that, he broke out into a long, loud laugh, one of those deep belly laughs that makes its way up the back of the throat and comes out hissing. "I give up," he said, laughing so hard he seemed to be crying. The laughter, of course, was broadcast throughout the park. When we finally found Arson, he was hopping mad, blaming us for "setting up" the announcer. No matter how much we denied it, Arson just couldn't believe we weren't involved. It took weeks before we could be buddies again.

We had found Arson by "Mr. Insult," one of the main attractions at Willow Grove. As you walked by, Mr. Insult would taunt you. "Hey you, yeah, you with the drool! Buy three balls. Come on, three balls for one lousy dime. See if you can hit the target and knock me in the water. Come on. Three balls. One lousy dime." If you didn't buy, Mr. Insult would step up the taunts. "Hey, hey, hey, is that an accident or is that your wife?" Or, "Hey, hey, hey, buddy, what'd you do to look that way? Take ugly pills?" "Hey, hey, hey, you ought to get a permit for that face, lady." Knowing us because we came so often, Mr. Insult would always shout out our special names. Johnnie was "Pimple Puss," Arson was "Hose Nose," Connie was "White Boy," and I—I was "Vomit Face."

Later I discovered Willow Grove had a dark side when I worked there one summer in the skills stands. You didn't get a regular salary. You made money by cheating the customers. Someone would be getting four dollars in change, and you'd count "one," then "two," but just before "three" you'd cough, distracting the customer while you picked up the second bill which then became the "third" dollar. If they caught you, you'd blame it on a cold, and ninety-nine times out of a hundred you'd get away with it.

One day on our way to the park John and I had stopped at Ormandy's grocery store and bought a pack of candy cigarettes. They looked real, with a red tip, but were just candy.

"From a distance you can't tell they're fake."

"Yeah, just like Dad's."

"It's the red tip that does it, right?"

"Right."

"Hey, Sid, let's go ride the Caterpillar and smoke these."

Now the Caterpillar was a long car that made a huge circle as it rode on a hilly track. When the ride started out, you sat in the open air, but about halfway through a top descended and then you were in the dark, going round and round, up and down, inside the caterpillar's belly. The older kids liked it because they made out underneath the cover.

John and I took the only two seats left, right in the center of the Caterpillar. As the ride started, John suggested, "Want a cigarette?" "Sure, man," I replied, imitating one of the teenagers. In a few minutes we were "smoking" away.

Suddenly the old man who operated the Caterpillar shouted, "Hey, you two boys there!" When we looked up, he continued, "Put that cigarette out."

Above the roar of the machinery I tried to tell him that we weren't smoking real cigarettes. But he couldn't hear and so once more shouted, "Put that cigarette out." And a third time, "Put that cigarette out."

John and I didn't want to cause any trouble and so we bit into the candy and swallowed it. Just as we did, a little boy sitting behind us began chanting, "Put that cigarette out. Put that cigarette out." The rhythm was two long beats, three short ones, followed by one long. On a piano the notes would be E E D B D E—going down and then up the scale.

"Put that cigarette out! Put that cigarette out."

Before I knew it, John and I were tapping our feet in rhythm, joining him: two longs on "Put that," three shorts for "cigarette," followed by a long "out." Soon the couple in front of us turned around, started to laugh, and joined in. The song, however stupid, now spread from row to row, so that by the time the Caterpillar top closed over us, everyone on the ride was singing, "Put that cigarette out." People outside heard a chorus of invisible people singing "Put that cigarette out." A catchy rhythm coming from a caterpillar's belly. When the ride was over, we all poured out, laughing and singing. We even shared our candy cigarettes. As our fellow riders departed, the song spread all over the park.

Every once in a while, for the rest of that evening, you'd hear someone in the park break out with a "Put that cigarette out" and then laugh. Old people, young people, teenagers, parents, children. Perfect strangers would look at each other, burst into grins, and salute with a "Put that cigarette out." People would play jokes on each other. "Hey, Bill, there's something I just have to tell you." Falling for it, Bill would ask, "What's that?" whereupon he'd get a "Put that cigarette out."

All the way home, my brother and I sang that silly refrain, playing variations on the rhythm, the notes, until we were sick of the song, promising each other not to sing it again and then double-crossing the other by breaking out with just one more "Put that cigarette out." It was several days before we got it out of our systems.

⁓#⁓

As the kids went back to their rooms they broke into impromptu choruses of "Put that cigarette out," some dancing to the silly rhythm, others, their heads together, imitating backup singers for the featured performer. Giving me a dirty look, the head nurse was clearly not pleased as they moved joyously down the hall, not just disturbing patients but mentioning the "c" word in a hospital that had long since banned cigarettes, not only in the buildings itself, or the lounges, but within two hundred feet of any entrance.

It seemed so long since that first day in Charlie's Corner when I met Tommy. Now he, all the patients, and their parents were part of my life, and, no less, I had become part of theirs.

"You're a hero to them," John Graham-Pole had said casually to me in the hallway the day before.

"Oh, come on, John. That's embarrassing . . . and just not true.

"I mean it, Sid."

"Hell, if anyone's a hero, it's you. You're their doctor. I'm just . . . I'm just an entertainer."

"Look, if it were just entertainment, a juggler would do, or one of those clowns who makes animals out of balloons."

"John, I help them escape for a while. You're the one who battles the cancer."

"Battles it, Sid, but never wins. I keep it at bay, hold it off for awhile, ease their pain. But it always wins." Then, after a pause he added, "Look, there are all sorts of heroes. You don't just entertain. I've seen them with you—and I've seen their parents. This world," and here he waved his hand to encompass the examination and operating rooms, the bedrooms of the Bone Marrow Unit, "this world here is closing in on them. Outside the hospital, their homes, might just as well be a million miles away. Invisible. Nothing exists for them but this unit. And it's a unit where the most desperate cases go . . . and where people die all the time. I know it, you know it—they know it. So, each Wednesday you bring that outside, real world to them, and they make it their own. Sid, they live through you. Your life, growing up in Philly, becomes their life. I know. When I make rounds, they're full of stories, some pretend, some real from whatever life they knew before they came here, and some plagiarized . . . that's the word . . . beautifully, wonderfully, humanly plagiarized from you. Sid, that's life-giving. That's the reason I started this Arts in Medicine Program. You were there when we founded the organization, when we had to justify it to the *hospital administrators. Artists can also be physicians, treating patients, concerned about their health. Helping save them from death, if only for a little while. That's all I do too, Sid, save them from death for a little while. So, my neurotic friend, there's all sorts of heroism."*

Tears, generous tears, came to my eyes.

"Now, give me a hug, and get home. By God, it's six already!"

"See you next Wednesday, John."

"Right-o," he replied in his crisp British way.

As I headed toward the parking lot, that word "hero" wouldn't go away. The hero with clay feet. Hero sandwich. The tragic hero. Hamlet. King Lear. Ordinary people who become heroes under emergent occasions. The ambiguous hero. The contradictory hero. Heroes who fall from grace. The hero as fool—the fool as hero. As I got into the car I thought of the mythic hero, the hero I envied, from my own high-school days. And of my favorite English teacher, who was caught in that same contradiction of hero and fool. **I Envied Harry Lewis** *would be my next story on Charlie's Corner.*

I envied Harry Lewis. Even his name. In high school girls fawned over him, and every guy hoped Harry would be his best buddy. Harry was perfect. Even when his hair was mussed, he still looked handsome. Yet there was nothing showy about Harry. He wasn't the quarterback on the football team; he didn't need to be. Actually, he was the tight end and one of the best players ever at that position in the history of the school. The most attractive girl in the class was Harry's girlfriend, about to be, or wanted to be. He moved about campus like an Adonis, with his best friend, Eddie Lipton, in attendance. Eddie was Harry's social secretary and his bodyguard, the guy you approached if you wanted to know whose party Harry was going to Saturday night. He *spoke* for Harry. As you might expect, Harry was a straight-A student, president of the senior class, and on Saturday mornings he volunteered at a nursing home.

No girl fawned over me; my buddies were a collection of misfits, rejected by everyone else as too smart, or freaky, or just plain different. Something was always doing at Harry's—a party, a political rally, neighbors dropping by with casseroles. Except for Mrs. Klecto coming over to borrow a cup of this or that, or an occasional visit from the Hanrahans—strange people whom my mother had taken under her wing after Mrs. Hanrahan reported that her husband beat her—no one came to our house, no one visited. When I was younger, this isolation was strangely comforting, part of my mother's conscious strategy to keep the world at arm's length. But in high school that outside world couldn't be denied. Harry was its prince, moving through the halls with grace and confidence, getting those looks from girls.

Saturday night I worked as a pantry boy at the Casa Argenio restaurant; Friday was family night, the gatherings around the radio giving way, without fanfare, to gatherings around the television. There was church Sunday morning. Beyond this, I had to scramble for a social life. What I usually wound up doing was cruising the streets of the city with my buddies, pressing our noses against the windows of parties to which we had not been invited but where Harry, visible in a crowd the way Hollywood movie stars stand out in street scenes, received all the attention—and was every girl's most ardent desire.

Harry even transformed his misfortunes into victories. The Abington-Cheltenham game was the high point of the baseball season. Harry was on the mound. Eddie Lipton was behind the plate. I was on the bench—as usual. As the batter hit Harry's very first pitch right back to the mound, Harry doubled over, cupping his hands in front of his pants, crying in pain. We all knew what had happened—that most embarrassing of all sports injuries. In a moment the team had made a circle around Harry, so that he could suffer in private, thereby maintaining his dignity. Now with any other player an accident like this, and on the first pitch, would have led to howls of laughter. With any other player there would have been rude jokes about manhood, double entendres, boys trying to top each other with put-downs and girls red in the face with embarrassment. Not in Harry's case. The crowd let up a cry of sympathy and concern. Ellen Smalley, Harry's girlfriend of the week, swooned; old or would-be girlfriends hugged each other. The next day Harry stayed home where he received calls and cards of sympathy, gifts from friends as well as perfect strangers. A bad pitch, a ridiculous hit to the groin, and yet when Harry returned to school two days later he was greeted like a war hero.

I envied the Harrys of this world. The darlings of fortune. I yearned for that intriguing, wild, exotic, unpredictable world where each day would be like Harry's days, full of friends, women, adventures, offers, invitations to accept or turn down, a parade of handsome people who made it through life effortlessly, favored, rewarded, a world where there was only success upon success. I envied Harry Lewis.

High school, at least, allowed me the illusion of being part of this swirl, this eddy of romance and adventure, rather than someone just sitting alone on the bench, watching Harry's teammates surround him as the girls in the stands wept over his wound. However imperfectly, high school would serve as something of a "practice" reality for me. Even there Harry dogged me every minute, for we had identical class schedules.

Our first class was Shop, held deep in the second basement, the domain of the feared Mr. Jantzen, a grizzled veteran of industry, slave master in a kingdom where no woman ever entered. His was a large, dank rectangular room of lathes, drill presses, and electric saws. Above Jantzen's desk, on a faded plaque, was his motto, "Good Men Make Good Goods." However illogical the assertion, here was the single, unalterable principle on which he conducted his classes, as well as established the scale on which there were only two points—"mother's boy" and "man." A man, Harry handled an electric saw indifferent to the fate of his fingers, indeed, winning Mr. Jantzen's fatherly approval by daring the saw as he held the board within millimeters of its whirling blades. A man like Harry breathed in the smell of sawdust or oil with style. A man used a ruler, a plane, or triangle with contempt. A mother's boy? I was a mother's boy. "You hold that nail like a damn baby holds a rattle!" Jantzen would bark at me. "What're ya afraid of, Homan? Think the saw's gonna kiss ya?" Trying to fashion a baseball bat on a spinning lathe, I cut in too deeply, the end product looking like some elongated toothpick. Sandpapering his bat, Harry meanwhile was on the verge of graduating to the next stage, applying the varnish. Jantzen grabbed my bat from the spinning lathe, smashed it against the back of a chair, and as it lay there in pieces on the shop floor bellowed, "There, ya mother's boy, clean up your 'D'!"

Second period Harry and I moved on to Miss Hirst, the art teacher with the hearing aid whose controls were just under the third button of her blouse. When the class got too loud, she would reach deep into her bosom to lower the volume. Speak in a whisper, and the hand shot again to her chest, not so artfully disguising the fact that she was turning the knob. As the class came into the art room one day, with Harry serving as ringleader, we mimed noises, "shouting" at each other but, in reality, only moving our lips and flailing our arms without a sound. One boy pretended to slam a stack of books on his desk but stopped just short of doing so. Someone else faked a loud, soundless argument within earshot of Miss Hirst. Thinking she had turned down the volume too low, the poor lady reached into her bosom. The moment Harry was sure the fateful knob had been adjusted, he gave the signal for us to scream and pound away. Clutching her hands to her ears, Miss Hirst let out a single cry and sank to her desk. The next day we had a substitute. Rumor had it that the entire class would have been suspended if Harry had not been involved.

Miss Lowrey was our high-school Latin teacher, and, as far as she was concerned, third-period Latin was the only legitimate subject we studied. She was a little woman, wiry, always in black, and had what we called a "lazy" eye, the right eyeball drifting towards her nose. To complicate things, she was blind in the left eye. So, in class when Miss Lowrey called on a student, she looked at a forty-five degree angle from where you were sitting, catching you from the side with her one good eye. Since no one wanted to offend Miss Lowrey—her temper was legendary—you had to figure out the trajectory of that misplaced right eye. If she looked directly at you, clearly it was not your turn to respond.

On Fridays each of us had to "take the bench," a seat at the front of the class with an armrest in front so that you slid into position from the left side. With Caesar's *Gallic Wars* or Ovid's *Ars Amores* held tightly in the right hand, you were to place your left on that armrest, knuckles up. Miss Lowrey stood to one side, brandishing a large ruler. When you made the slightest mistake in translation—pluperfect for perfect, or ablative for genitive—no matter how minor the mistake, she would whack the offending knuckles with that ruler. You would learn Latin Miss Lowrey's way or else, since, for her, all the achievements of Western civilization were mere afterthoughts, spokes on a wheel whose core was ancient Rome. Harry was her favorite and the only one who never had his knuckles cracked. Once she told him in her youth the Hollywood director, Cecil B. DeMille, had been her lover.

William Kerrigan Esser, the history teacher in fourth period, had blackboards stretching from floor to ceiling on all four walls of his windowless room. Immediately behind his desk were the names of every student in his classes. His wife, a short, chubby woman, her pockmarked face in a perpetual sneer, manned the boards, a piece of chalk ready in her left hand, her right controlling a ladder like the type you find in libraries or bookstores, reaching to the ceiling and connected there by castors, with nine steps up which she would scurry to make entries. Using a system so complex that no student had ever fathomed it, Mr. Esser would award or subtract points depending on your "performance" in class. Get the right answer to a question and he would order Mrs. Esser to enter a "5" by your name. A subsequent wrong answer brought a "–3" after that "5," with a "5" and an additional "2" (his or her reward for making the correction) going by the name of the classmate coming up with the right answer. Improve on a classmate's answer and, for some inexplicable reason, you'd get not only a "5" but an additional "5," while your classmate lost all five points. If you asked an impromptu question that stumped a fellow student, you were given 20 points. Misbehave and you lost points, the sliding scale going from "–2" for an uncovered sneeze to a "–100"— this was the record—to Arthur Frank when he hurled a book across the room and hit Eddie McShane in the left temple. Make an intelligent point, ask an appropriate question, and reward followed. Say something stupid or irrelevant, and Mrs. Esser, like an owl spotting a mouse scurrying towards its hole, would find your name and, with a gleeful hissing of her breath, subtract points. The scoring changed day to day, without pattern. Generally, right answers got more points towards the end of the week, yet this was not always the case.

Mr. Esser seemed especially to value improving on a classmate's answer, even more than correcting someone else, yet we all recalled that glorious first week in February when correcting got twice as many points as improving. Bonuses came, albeit rarely, like bolts out of the blue. "Give Parham an extra six points," he once said to Mrs. Esser, never addressing her by name. A pleasant enough girl, but totally silent in class, near the bottom of the point total, Marla Parham got her bonus without apparent rhyme or reason. "That Winer kid, minus ten," Mr. Esser called out one day, and for the rest of the week we all puzzled over what Alfie's infraction had been—an inadvertent sneeze that somehow Mrs. Esser, who never missed such things, had failed to record earlier? Or had Alfie possibly looked the wrong way, slurred a syllable, or come to school with a spot on his shirt?

As you might imagine, there were no discipline problems in Mr. Esser's class. Our attention was focused on gaining points, on not losing points, and on watching Mrs. Esser race up and down the ladder, making entries, pushing the ladder forward and backwards, a whirl of activity, her only break being between classes. Even then she never left the room, never left her station, but rather stayed by her ladder like some patient sentry. We were all neurotic in Mr. Esser's class, caught between joy and sorrow as our point total rose and fell, sometimes with good reason, sometimes without apparent cause or explanation. To make matters worse, Mr. Esser graded on a curve, and so we were in direct competition with each other, the aristocracy at the top determining the coveted A, the rest of us sealing our own mediocrity by clustering our score near the center of Esser's curve.

Mr. Esser himself was something of a marionette, sporting colorful "English" ties and well-cut jackets, his face fashionably pale. He spoke in a precise way that bordered on affectation. Until my senior year, Mrs. Esser never spoke. We speculated she was mute, overburdened with some dark past, or that speaking even a single word, a vowel, would somehow compromise her position as her husband's faithful recorder. The only time she spoke was the day Joan Case challenged Mr. Esser's system. Well, not so much challenged it as demanded an explanation of the rationale of rewards and punishments, or the relation between points in a single category, like—say—social indiscretions or clever retorts. Actually, Joan's challenge took the form of a simple and, in its way, profound announcement. Rising from her seat and walking partly down the row towards Mr. Esser's desk, as if to meet him halfway on the matter, she exclaimed, "Mr. Esser, your system is unfair." He looked at Joan for the longest time, his expression that of a hurt bird. Then he turned to Mrs. Esser. Her face full of compassion, the first emotion we had ever seen her register, she walked over to her husband, actually *left* the ladder, and put her right hand on his shoulder. Another first, for although we knew they were married, we had never seen the slightest trace of affection between them. His hurt expression dissolving, Mr. Esser began searching the air with his eyes for the proper response to Joan's challenge. At last, looking at Joan directly, with a penetrating glance, he replied, "Miss Case, *life* is unfair." For the first and only time Mrs. Esser spoke. Clasping her husband's shoulder more tightly, as if that earlier gesture of affection, however slight, had now changed to conviction, she uttered a simple "Yes." A "yes" coming from deep inside her soul, a "yes," one somehow felt, having little to do with Joan's challenge, a "yes" speaking volumes about the poor woman's silence, a silence, we speculated, born out of fate's shabby, capricious treatment of her. A final first: her sneer changed, though for just a brief moment, to a grin.

With that, it was back to the ladder. As if he had been cleansed by his answer to Joan, Mr. Esser joyfully announced, "Ten points and an additional fifteen bonus points to anyone who can give me the name of the Roman senator who ended every speech he gave in the Forum, no matter what the topic, with the sentence, "Censeo Karthaginem esse delendam." Having just heard Miss Lowrey refer to the line in Latin class, I put up my hand.

"Yes?"

Trying to get extra points I decided to embellish my answer. "It was Cato the Younger and, by the way, the translation is, "I vote that we destroy Carthage."

Harry Lewis's hand shot up. "No, it was Cato the Elder."

"Take three points from the Homan boy for the wrong answer, plus give eight points to Mr. Lewis for the right answer and for correcting him." Just when I thought my humiliation was through, Mr. Esser added, "And deduct an extra two points from Homan."

"Why, Mr. Esser?" I blurted out.

"Your translation was irrelevant to the question."

Life is unfair.

Final period we had Mr. Gessner for English. We loved him. A bald man, with eyes announcing that everything about the world and everything about his students fascinated him, with a walk like that of a cowboy sauntering about the ranch, with a voice rich and deep, a voice that caressed words before handing them over to the listener, he conducted classes as if he were the local bartender and you were customers coming in for a drink and a chat. Class never formally started or ended. You showed up as soon as possible, spent the time discussing literature, your visit cruelly cut short by the bells on which other mediocre teachers so depended. Because his class was so informal, his style so casual, we nicknamed Mr. Gessner "The Friendly Bartender." He laughed every time we called him that.

The semester assignment listed ten novels, classics like Conrad's *Victory*, Fitzgerald's *Tender Is the Night*, and Austen's *Pride and Prejudice*. We were to hand in five one-thousand word essays, but at any time we wanted and on any topic falling within the confines of that reading list. Mr. Gessner asked questions, but not about the novel's "meaning" or "theme." He had an aversion to words like "theme," telling us he found them too limiting, arguing that a novel is a moment-by-moment experience, a "transaction" between the writer and the reader.

"If I should ever mention 'theme' in class, I'll give a dollar to the first person who catches me doing it." He never had to pay up.

Mr. Gessner's questions would center on what you were feeling, experiencing, or thinking about, line by line, moment by moment in the novel. Or, why the character said what he said. "What's he after with that question?" "What's his object?" Mr. Gessner asked us to suspend disbelief and see characters as real people, with objects, desires, and agendas both known and unknown to them. "What's happening, what's going on?" In The Friendly Bartender's class it was unthinkable not to have a novel read in time, or to come to those daily conversations unprepared. Writing more than a thousand words on a paper, or handing in an extra assignment—these were never put down as trying to brownnose.

We learned from Ellie Sullivan, whose mother was the principal's secretary, that once at a faculty meeting some of the teachers complained to the principal that Mr. Gessner was giving too many A's, that his grades were thirty percent above the school average. "How can the same student who makes a C in my class legitimately get an A in yours?" Mr. Marks, the Civics teacher, demanded—again, all this as reported by Ellie. Apparently, Mr. Gessner replied that indeed the student might deserve a C in Mr. Marks's class, in fact, might even earn a B from "such an average teacher." But in his class that same student, he said, became "better than her normal self, discovered all sorts of hidden talents," and that the A he gave, therefore, was logical, in fact, "probably a bit lower than she actually deserved." With the principal leading the charge, the faculty found him "out of order," "insulting," and "arrogant." Endlessly repeating Mr. Gessner's words in conversations at lunchtime and in the halls, we kids treated them as if they were from a sacred text, words that made life more bearable as we suffered through those pedestrian teachers on the first floor. Those words, as reported by Ellie, were my touchstone in the subterranean classroom of Mr. Jantzen as he screamed at me for cutting an irregular pair of bookends.

The week before school ended for the spring semester, Mr. Gessner invited the seniors in his advanced literature course to dinner at his house. We were to arrive at seven. That invitation was the big news, our chance to see how this godlike figure, our hero, lived, to meet his wife. When Harry Lewis suggested we buy him a gift, we held a meeting and all decided to arrive all at the same time. To surprise Mr. Gessner we would have our parents drop us off early a block from his house. Then, at five of seven we would assemble on his lawn and, precisely on the hour, knock on the door. When he opened the door, as a single voice we would shout, "We love you, friendly bartender." Harry Lewis was chosen—*of course*—to hand Mr. Gessner the gift, a handsome copy of the *Oxford English Dictionary* and a bouquet of roses.

Everything went according to plan. To make sure we knocked right on schedule and that everyone was properly arranged on the front lawn so that the "friendly bartender" line would come off perfectly, we started walking to his house earlier than planned, figuring an extra five minutes would provide a margin of safety.

As we got to Mr. Gessner's house at about ten to seven, though, we heard angry voices coming from inside. Mr. Gessner and his wife were screaming, calling each other all sorts of names. Charges were traded back and forth.

"You don't think I know what you've been doing?"

"You dumb slut, what the hell do you know about anything!"

"Slut? How dare you, you goddamn lush."

"Lush? Look's who's calling who a lush?"

The woman's cry "Don't you!" led to the sound of someone being hit, and then the blow returned. Weeping accompanied a crash as if a chair had been knocked over. Suddenly Mr. Gessner shouted, "God, it's almost seven!"

Harry Lewis looked at me, "Sid, what should we do?" With my hands, with no need or time for words, I suggested we go ahead as planned. In a flash we were arranged in formation on the lawn. With a desperate "Here, I can't do it," Harry handed me the gift and the flowers as Alan Schmidt knocked on the door. In ten seconds or so, it opened and there stood the Gessners, their pose suggesting they were the happiest of couples. Mr. Gessner even had his arm around his wife. With our best faces possible, we screamed, "We love you, friendly bartender!" and if some of us cried, feeling the irony of that line now that this darker side of our hero had been inadvertently exposed, such crying actually helped the illusion, as if the tears were those of joy, of love. In one sense, they were. Mr. Gessner himself cried as he accepted the gift.

We were engaging guests, hiding our secret from the Gessners who, clearly, playing the gracious hosts, thought they were hiding a secret from us.

We took no pleasure in pretending that nothing had happened. Yet the evening also went quickly, for in a curious way it was exhilarating keeping up the pretense. I felt like a character in one of those novels we read in Mr. Gessner's classes, or an actor playing a part and yet also being my real self, a student shocked that his teacher, this man of such elegant words, could be so woefully human.

Mercifully, the evening was soon over. Once outside, Harry Lewis came up to me and said, "Thanks, Sid, for knowing what to do. I was lost. I'm glad you were there." The perfect one, Harry Lewis was thanking me!

My buddy Connie Armbruster asked me to spend the night. Lying on the floor, our feet propped against the wall and looking out his bedroom window at the cloudy night sky, we went over the details of the evening. We wished desperately that we could preserve Mr. Gessner as the teacher we knew at school, as our hero The Friendly Bartender.

"How can we face him on Monday?"

"He doesn't know that we know."

"Sure, but *we* know."

"We'll handle it. I mean, he's not suddenly going to become a bad teacher, like the rest of them."

"But it won't be the same."

"You're right there."

Then, after a long silence, I added, "What did we expect, Connie? That he'd be perfect at home too?"

As I lay in bed I thought of Mr. Gessner. And then of Conrad's *Victory*. My beloved teacher had told us the journey was a basic motif in literature. More than going to a new place, the journey was a voyage into one's self. "When you leave what has become familiar and comfortable, when you leave home, you abandon your old self. When you arrive at your destination, you are not the same person who left." He had added, "This is a cause neither for sadness nor for unwarranted optimism."

Just before I fell asleep Harry Lewis came to my mind. Why had he asked me, *me* of all the kids there on the lawn, what we should do? And why had he handed me, *me* the gift and the flowers to present to The Friendly Bartender? There were others he knew better. Others just as able, probably more so, to make a decision. Why hadn't Harry himself made the decision, Harry, president of the senior class, starting tight end on the football team, Harry Lewis, the guy I envied?

Fifteen years later, I met Harry Lewis at the only high-school reunion I ever attended. Potbellied and drunk, he staggered into the men's room, where he tried to entertain us by making crude jokes about his wife.

CHAPTER 12

The Ever-Present

Remembering what John Graham-Pole had said about my role as storyteller, I decided to try once more to confront that subject of death ever-present in the Bone Marrow Unit. Today, without asking the teenagers for a subject, breaking the ritualistic "Have you heard?" or "Did I ever tell you about?" I launched right away into **It's Bootiful**.

⟨⸻⟩

My grandfather was the first licensed electrician in Philadelphia, and he wisely used the money he earned to buy row houses all along Broad Street. As a result, he was our only wealthy relative. Of the sixty-one members of our family living in or near the city, or upstate, not one of them liked Grandfather. But they all wanted his money. Except me. I didn't care about the money; I found Grandfather fascinating.

A Cockney, with a tough, working-class British accent, he was a round man, short and very powerful. Even in his seventies, he could take a heavy ax, the type workers use to dig up roadways, and hold it straight out with one arm, without a trace of shaking. He always had a stubble of beard, and his hands smelled of electrical tape. Grandfather cursed all the time, much to the dismay of my grandmother who, unlike him, had come from a polite English family and spoke in a proper, upper-class style.

Refined, never given to saying anything directly, most at home serving tea and plum pudding every afternoon, Grandmother had married a crude man, direct, full of opinions on everything. On Grandfather's desk was a stone paperweight he claimed was the petrified tongue of a German soldier he had "killed for the Queen" in World War I.

Grandmother never, ever entered the basement, for that was Grandfather's workshop, row after row of shelves on which was arranged in perfect order the equipment of a lifetime, everything an electrician would ever need. Grandfather used to let my brother John and me explore down there. The workshop had an earthen floor. In one corner stood a coal bin and a huge furnace that looked like an octopus with its "arms" rising into the ceiling to carry heat to the five apartments in the building.

Though he never told me, I knew Grandfather was disappointed in his stepson, my father. Partly for the fact that Dad got TB as a child, a sign of weakness in Grandfather's view of things. But mostly because Dad had married, for it was clear Grandfather did not like my mother.

Mother was very socially conscious; she did everything she could to escape her blue-collar family. She married my father for love, I am sure, but also because he had a nice English last name, Homan. My mother's maiden name was Polish, Cyrnereski—"too Polish" I once heard her say. Without going through any legal process, mother had unofficially changed her first name, Mary, to May Elaine. For her, Mary called up the Virgin Mary and the Catholic Church of her youth; May Elaine sounded English and Episcopalian. My father, whatever he was not, was a member of that church, a "proper church" in my mother's opinion.

We lived in a working-class district of the city, but Mother, knowing that wealthy people had artwork in their homes, bought one of those large mass-produced paintings from the Five and Dime and, in the lower right-hand corner, wrote the name of a fictitious artist—D. L. Drew. Soon, our house was covered with the works of this mythical D. L. Drew. "Whistler's Mother" was now by D. L. Drew, as was Van Gogh's "Sunflower" and—for good measure—that Turner painting of a man in a rowboat surrounded by an angry sea.

Now, Grandfather was also an artist, a very fine one, though he claimed to paint landscapes only to cover "the [and here he would curse] cracks in the walls." One night at dinner he laughed at my mother for inventing D. L. Drew, and relations between them, which had always been formal, now chilled even further.

Like the other sixty-one members of the family, except me— and I would have to add my father and brother—my mother wanted Grandfather's money. Rumor was that he had "salted away about two million." These were Aunt Grace's words. She wanted his money too, as did Uncle Eddie and Aunt Marie and Aunt Francis and everyone else. So, even after his attack on D. L. Drew, Mother still called every Friday night to invite Grandmother and Grandfather to dinner on Saturday. At the table, she would pretend that everything was fine, complimenting the old man about this and that, acting as if his gruff answers were, instead, courteous, elegant prose. My grandfather knew that my mother knew that he knew that she knew—and so on forever—just why she was being so polite.

Five weeks after the D. L. Drew episode, Grandfather took his revenge on her. At the end of the meal the custom at our house was to serve mincemeat pie, Grandfather's favorite, and, adding custom on custom, Grandfather always cut the first piece for himself, then passed the pie to my mother to serve the rest of the family.

Biting her tongue, casting looks at my father, all the while telling my grandfather how "perfectly delighted" she was to have him for dinner, Mother passed the pie dish over to the old man. Carefully watching her the whole time, Grandfather cut a modest wedge in the pie. Mother handed him a plate on which to put that modest wedge. Now, with one eye on her and the other on the pie, Grandfather proceeded to lift the rest of the pie from its dish—that is, about eighty percent or a clock from twelve to ten—putting it instead on his plate. Then, pushing the dish with the wedge towards my mother, he said, "There, Mary [not the usual May Elaine], I leave the rest of the pie to you and the family. Homans, enjoy your pie." Mother could barely refrain from giving him a piece of her mind and risk being disinherited. Normally the boss of our family, Mother caved in and, with Grandmother as usual refusing a piece, divided the sliver among the four of us. Grandfather patted my hand under the table.

Grandfather *was* a character; *everyone* in town knew him. There were many legends about the old man, many started by Grandfather himself. About how every morning when he woke from his Murphy bed, one of those beds you pull out from the wall, he would drink a half-bottle of gin before he got up. When I walked the streets of Philadelphia with him, going to check on his row houses, people would stop to tell my grandfather the neighborhood news, to ask his view of the latest controversy, to laugh or blush at his risqué jokes.

On Friday afternoons, after tea, Grandfather and I would sit on the front porch of his row house, greeting neighbors as they passed by. One afternoon we were doing just that when Mrs. Everett, who lived five houses up Broad Street, came by with her poodle.

"Good afternoon, Mrs. Everett," my grandfather said politely. Of course, I repeated what he said.

"Lovely day," she replied, "And I see you have young Master Sidney with you."

My grandfather began to chat with Mrs. Everett, but as he did, her dog pulled a bit at his leash. Mrs. Everett saw him yet went on talking. The dog pulled again, and a second time she ignored him. Finally, the dog went into action and made "a little deposit" right in the middle of my grandfather's miniature lawn. Grandfather saw it from the corner of his eye, yet went right on with the conversation, acting as if he hadn't. I was watching the whole time. I saw Mrs. Everett see what her dog did, and I also saw her see my grandfather see what the dog did. Besides seeing him see that she saw what the dog did, she saw that I saw what the dog did. Everybody saw everybody else see what the dog did. I don't know what the dog saw, or didn't see.

Shortly after the dog did what we all saw, Mrs. Everett, a little flustered, said good-bye and continued down the street as if nothing had happened. After a minute, my grandfather stroked his chin and then, turning to me, announced, "Sidney, I think I have a little present for Mrs. Everett. Follow me."

He went to the backyard, got a small shovel, then returned to the apartment and found a shoebox. Going back to the lawn, grandfather scooped up the "deposit," dropped it in the box, and replaced the lid. Then he turned the box upside down, wrapped it in bright paper, and tied a ribbon around it so that it looked like a gift. Putting on his hat, he said, "Shall we pay a visit to Mrs. Everett?" I couldn't wait.

A few minutes later we rang her doorbell.

"Well, what a delightful surprise, Mr. Homan," and then, right on cue, she added, "And Master Sidney. Do come in."

My grandfather walked to the center of her living room, stopped, and handed Mrs. Everett the "present."

"What . . . what is this?" she asked, all alive with curiosity.

"Madam, earlier today you gave me a little surprise, a present, you might say. Now I'd like to return the favor."

Mrs. Everett didn't get it, hadn't a clue, but, instead, broke into a big smile, practically grabbing the box from the old man.

"A present! A present for me! How delightful!" she cried to herself as she tore into the wrapping paper. No longer held in place, the lid on the bottom fell to the floor; a split second afterwards the deposit landed right in the middle of the carpet. Mrs. Everett shrieked.

Walking back up Broad Street was exhilarating, and I knew my grandfather was enjoying it too because, normally a tight-wad, he stopped at an ice-cream store and bought me a double-decker.

And Grandfather would strike again later that day. This time a different woman was involved.

When she heard about the episode with the dog, Mother complained that he'd ruined her appetite for the church oyster supper that night. A big event in the neighborhood, the supper raised money for the missionary fund. There was always some sort of entertainment in the parish hall afterwards.

Mother was in charge of both the dinner and the entertainment. In the kitchen crews prepared the oysters in huge vats of fat; others cooked vegetables or sliced pies for dessert. Mother organized servers and greeters and cleaners. I was put on the dishwashing crew. So many people were involved in preparing and serving the supper that there was really no one left in the church to be the guests, or "customers." So the parishioners played both roles—eating and serving, serving and eating. In the center of everything, my mother barked orders like a captain on the deck of a ship, her crew obedient and diligent.

That Friday night Mother had hired a hypnotist for the after-dinner entertainment. When everyone had assembled in the parish hall, he asked for volunteers. My grandfather joined seven other audience members onstage. Within a few minutes, swinging a pendant on a chain and talking in a monotone, the hypnotist had put all eight to sleep.

"When I snap my fingers once, you will wake up and remember nothing. When I snap my fingers twice you will fall back into a deep sleep where you will hear only my voice."

One snap and his subjects woke up. During some polite conversation with him, none showed any signs of knowing that they had been asleep just minutes before. Two snaps and instantly the eight went back into a trance, their heads lowered on their chests, their eyes glassy. Then, one by one, the hypnotist asked the volunteers to tell about their most pleasant experience when they were young. An older man recounted his first date; a woman described the swing on which she used to play with her sister; a third told about the best meal he had ever had; another, a birthday party she attended when she was five. Each relived the past, sometimes talking in a child's voice, showing by their expressions that, for them, the experience was happening all over again. They were excited, full of joy, and as uninhibited as they had been stiff, even nervous onstage before.

The hypnotist then asked my grandfather the same question. There was a silence, as if the old man were traveling back in time, back over seventy years. Then, in a firm voice he began to describe a bathhouse in the suburb of London where he was born. It was a marvelous account—the streets, the flower sellers, the marble steps leading to the bathhouse, the dress of the people as they passed by. Next he took us into the interior of the bathhouse—the cashier at the far end of the lobby, the corridors to the changing rooms, the communal pool, the showers, the steam rooms. As he talked, his body, though now showing the first signs of arthritis, seemed to grow firm; dulled by years of living in this country, his Cockney accent returned until at times we strained to understand him.

Like a sleepwalker, he rose from his chair to address the audience as he recalled going to that bathhouse as a seventeen-year-old boy. After paying the cashier, he went to the changing room. Once undressed, a towel draped over his shoulder, he proceeded towards the pool, located inside an ornate wing of the bathhouse built during the reign of Queen Victoria. At first the pool appeared to be empty and he relished the thought of having it all to himself. Then, at the far end he saw a figure. A woman, bathing. She was naked! However, instead of turning modestly away from my grandfather, she beckoned, inviting him to come to her. He began to describe her body in graphic detail.

I couldn't hear what Grandfather said next because the parish hall broke into an uproar of laughter, shock, alarm. The hypnotist raced over to stop the old man but was pushed off rudely by that same arm capable of lifting an ax. The minister came onstage. To no avail. Grandfather got louder, his description of the encounter with the naked woman delivered in every gross detail. Amid all the confusion the audience would occasionally catch a word, an explicit adjective or verb, to be met with amusement or embarrassment.

Finally, coming onstage, Grandmother crossed over to the old man, and as she did the crowd became still. Very simply, in her perfect, upper-class British accent, she advised him, "Frederick, that is *quite* enough." He changed to a lamb. The hypnotist came up and snapped his finger once. Now fully awake and escorted by my grandmother, Grandfather left the stage. Just as things were returning to normal, we discovered that during all the excitement Mother had fainted. Whether out of shock or anger, I do not know. We were never allowed to discuss the evening. It was a silent, tense ride home in the car that night.

My grandfather's main passion proved inseparable from his death. Until his arthritis got serious and he was forced to enter a hospital for treatment, he would go once a year during the third week of December to Florida. During that week Grandfather would spend almost all of his time at the dog tracks. He bet modest amounts, to be sure, but bet he did. In the meanwhile, Grandmother visited friends who had retired there. On the way to Florida, Grandfather would drive his '50 Ford coupe at breakneck speeds, boasting, when he came home, of the numerous tickets he had collected.

Nothing could prevent this annual migration. In fact, to insure that he would be in the best of health for that third week in December and so wouldn't miss a single race at any of the six dog tracks, Grandfather would purposely give himself a cold at the start of December. His theory was that getting the cold "out of the way" before the trip allowed his system to build up antibodies, a guarantee that he would be healthy for Florida. So, during that first week of December he would stroll down Broad Street in his shorts, with the flimsiest of shirts, inviting the cold to attack him.

In his one-hundredth year, two weeks after he had returned from the dog tracks, my grandfather died. He was vigorous almost until the end. In fact, on the day he died we sat, as usual, on his front porch, acknowledging the greetings of neighbors passing by, sharing the small talk that at once defines and unites a neighborhood. By this time Grandfather's arthritis was painful, and as I helped him from his chair, I heard a slight cry from somewhere deep inside his chest. Still alert, he saw my reaction and, tightening his grip on me with the same hand that, just a few years before, could have lifted an ax, he said, "It's been bootiful, Sidney, bootiful." "Bootiful" was how my grandfather with his Cockney accent pronounced "beautiful."

As I placed his head gently on a pillow, his body stiffened and then he died. Curiously, a few seconds later he gave a sigh, like a word issuing from the mouth after the heart itself has stopped. I would learn later that the sound was not uncommon, that it came from air trapped in the lungs forcing its way out. I looked at him, the first licensed electrician in Philadelphia, his hands still smelling of tape, the face awash in the gray stubble of his beard. On the table lay the petrified tongue of the German solder he had killed eighty years before.

The long-awaited reading of Grandfather's will brought all sixty-one relatives to the lawyer's office. They sat surrounding him, eager to hear how much of Grandfather's reported two million dollars would be theirs.

"I, being of sound mind and body, leave sufficient funds, as arranged beforehand with my executor, to my widow, Alice, to attend to her needs for her remaining days."

The expected opening seemed reasonable to everyone, even to my mother who, I knew, was reliving those hundreds of Saturday dinners, especially Grandfather's "Homans, I leave you to your pie."

"To the Temple University School of Medicine, who cared so well for me, I leave the sum of one million dollars."

This was and was not a surprise. After all, that's where he had been treated for his arthritis. There was a polite, though slightly agitated murmur among the crowd as my relatives silently subtracted that amount from the reported two million.

Then came the shocker. "To the following six dog tracks in Florida, where I spent so many happy days—the Miami Beach Kennel Club [and here the lawyer proceeded to read the other five names]—I leave one million dollars for the perpetual upkeep of the floral displays and landscaping that make those places so beautiful." It was almost as if I could hear him say "bootiful." Panic spread among the survivors.

The two million gone! Cries of anguish, disbelief, half-articulated phrases about "the crazy old man" rang out. In his agitation, one Homan relative overturned a chair. Another slumped against the back wall with a loud thud. My mother stood half-crazed in the center of her relatives, beyond speech, knowing now that her years of patient suffering had been fruitless. Banging on the table with his fists, on the fifth try the lawyer restored order.

"Ladies and gentlemen. The will is not complete . . . the will is *not* complete."

But the two million was already gone? Did he have a third million salted away somewhere? Were there conditions to be imposed on the dog tracks? On the hospital? Curiosity, a touch of hope, desperation—all three, in some inexplicable combination, served more than the lawyer's plea to restore order. Seats were righted, hairdos rearranged, people took their places pretending that nothing had happened. For a few minutes the room had the decorum that greeted the earlier clause about my grandmother's welfare.

"To my beloved grandson, Sidney, I leave the sum of two hundred dollars." My cousin Grace, who would later become a professional softball player, pinched my cheek, and there was a general murmur of congratulations. Were the other sixty relatives now expecting two hundred dollars each? After all, two hundred dollars would be better than nothing.

For five years the family would contest the will, but Grandfather had outsmarted them all in the one clause that remained.

"And to the rest of the family, sixty in all, I leave each one the princely sum of *one dollar.*"

One month later I received the two hundred dollars. I never spent it. It is my own bootiful talisman.

CHAPTER 13

Tommy's Girlfriend

The next week in Charlie's Corner Tommy came in before the other kids. He confessed that he was sweet on Edna, Amanda's friend.

"I just want to know what . . . you know . . . you know, people your age did back then. Did you have a girlfriend?"

I was happy to oblige, and so I asked, "Did I ever tell you about **The Smartest Girl in the Class***?"*

For a glorious six months in my senior year, Alison Price, the smartest girl in the class, was my girlfriend. She was my first real date. Three days after I got my driver's license I asked her if I could take her to the movies in our four-door black 1938 Dodge. The car was bought to celebrate my birth; my parents saw no reason to replace it. But in 1956 it was humiliating to drive to Alison's house in that 1938 Dodge, black, with running boards, with a hood that opened in two halves like the wings of a bird, and a back trunk shaped like a woman's bustle. All the other guys were behind Chevys and Mercs, cars without running boards, cars that didn't look like hearses, cars that were modern.

Alison didn't care. This was her first date too. Skinny, no breasts, dull brown stringy hair, her body mannish, she had a rectangular face, and yet she moved her hands so gently, so carefully. Not a pretty girl, not the type you were supposed to take on a date, nevertheless I found her appealing. With a DA haircut that didn't quite make it in the back and more than my share of pimples, I was no great catch either. Still, Alison was a girl, and I'd bet she was also saying about me, "Still, he's a boy."

Alison's mother was easy to talk to; it was her father who terrified me. When he did speak he reminded me that "Alison has to be in by ten." I tried to impress him by promising that I would have her home fifteen minutes early. He was not impressed. Both parents perched in the doorway as we walked to the car. I had let Alison in the passenger's side and was going around the car when Mr. Price came down the steps towards me. Another reminder, I feared. "Great car, Sidney [he actually called me Sidney]. I had one of these myself, years ago. Runs for a million miles, great car—don't build them like that anymore." Suddenly, the black Dodge looked wonderful. As Mr. Price walked back towards his wife, however, he added, "Don't forget, young man—nine forty-five." With Alison smelling of lilacs, I backed out the drive.

We rode in silence until we were about five blocks from the theatre. I had to pull out onto a busy street, and couldn't see clearly out the passenger side because of all the cars double-parked. "Alison, do you see any cars coming that way?" I asked, waving my hand in her direction while checking out the traffic on my left.

"No, there's no cars coming," she said.

Just as I turned left onto Vine Street, a huge truck came bearing down from Alison's direction. As the truck swerved into the right lane to avoid hitting us, the driver cursed at me. I started shaking; Alison was blushing.

"Why didn't you tell me that truck was coming?"

"You only asked about cars, Sid—not trucks."

Maybe Alison wasn't so smart after all. Still, she was a girl.

"You know, come to think of it—you're right. I didn't."

Cheeks still red, she looked up at me. "Thanks."

We laughed. There was a lot in that "thanks," for from that moment on Alison and I discovered we had plenty to talk about.

We sat in the front of the theatre. Alison had suggested we share some popcorn; our hands touched as we reached into the bag. We both timed it so that we always went for more popcorn together. A senior two rows in front of us had his arm around his girl. I couldn't work up the nerve to do that with Alison. Besides, the bag of popcorn was serving nicely. Halfway through the movie the senior got up to go into the lobby, and just a few seconds after he was gone, a new boy sat down beside the girl. In a flash they were kissing, *really* kissing—they were making out! Less than a minute after the second guy left, the first guy returned with a new bag of popcorn. The girl greeted him as if nothing had happened. I looked at Alison; she smiled back at me.

The movie ended at 9:30. We had exactly fifteen minutes to make that self-imposed deadline I had promised Mr. Price. As we drove, we both became quiet once again. I don't know what Alison was thinking. I know what I was: Should I try to kiss her goodnight? As we walked towards her front porch, we could see her folks in the living room, pretending to watch television but, of course, really waiting for Alison to come inside. I wanted to kiss her.

"I had a great time."

"So did I, a *really* great time." Alison's "really" gave me some encouragement. I moved closer; she didn't move away. Then, for some stupid reason, I started to shake her hand, pumping it up and down the way my Uncle Eddie used to pump mine after a few drinks. Dumb words came from me that, the moment they were out of my mouth, I couldn't believe I had said. "Alison, I'd like to kiss you but, seeing that this is our first date, I don't think it would be proper. Don't you agree?"

Helpless, a bit crushed, she replied, "Of course," and turned away.

There was no way out, no way to take it back. Embarrassed, humiliated, most of all furious at myself, I started towards the car. Suddenly, I felt Alison's hand touching my right shoulder. She spun me around, put both arms around my waist, and kissed me. I mean *kissed* me. I could see Mr. Price bolt from his chair, his wife trying to restrain him. In a second I was in the

Dodge, backing out of the driveway. The father stood outlined in the front door. Mrs. Price, her hands on her hips, remained in the center of the living room.

Graduating first and second in our class, Alison and I had been picked to give commencement speeches just before the principal handed out diplomas. On a stage in the center of the football field, surrounded by hundreds of fellow students and their parents, Alison and I sat to one side towards the back, a huge American flag hanging from a pole between us. There was a strong wind that night, and as I waited to give my speech, I gallantly held the flag with my left hand so that it wouldn't flap in Alison's face. The wind was so strong that it was all I could do to hold that flag in place.

As skinny as ever, Alison still had no breasts. Yet I loved her, despite the fact that my friends nicknamed her "Flat Brain." For me, she was Alison who didn't tell me the truck was coming, Alison whose hand I had touched in the popcorn bag, Alison who had kissed me that first date despite my fumbling efforts.

After Alison came back to her chair, I got up to give my speech. As she whispered "good luck" to me with her eyes, I realized there would be a problem: Who would hold the flag for her? As Alison grabbed the end tightly in her right hand, she said, "Don't worry, Sid. I'll be OK. Don't worry." When I got to the lectern, I could feel the wind picking up. People in the audience started bundling themselves in their coats. Behind me I could hear that flag flapping wildly, like a whip being snapped. I began my speech.

"Sid! Help!"

I turned around just in time to see Alison, chair and all, caught up in the flag, flung to the football field five feet below the back of the stage. A crowd had already formed by the time I got to her. She was laughing! We all were. There was Alison, flat on her back, wrapped like a mummy in the American flag. "I'm sorry I ruined your speech, Sid," she whispered. I hugged her even tighter. I could see her mother smiling at us; her father, as usual, glared away.

That fall, I became a freshman at Princeton University. Alison went to Smith College. We knew we wouldn't meet again until Christmas vacation. Two months after the semester started, the girls in her dorm found Alison dead of alcohol poisoning.

⁓⚜⁓

"I didn't know that about you. That was good."

I patted Tommy on the head, and while he pretended to dismiss the gesture as "babyish," I knew he didn't really object. I had patted him on the head just the way my dear father used to.

I had also experimented with another story involving death and, despite Tommy's compliment, knew that the ending had affected him and the others who this day were my audience. John had been too kind, but wrong, in calling me a hero. But he was right in one respect: I was not just an entertainer. I was trying, in my own way and with what resources I had, to help the patients deal with their cancer, to put it in perspective. My stories, my performances, were not hermetically sealed, divorced from the real world. Even if I tried to make them so, my audience would not let them so remain.

What I was doing in Charlie's Corner began to influence my own work in the classroom and in the theatre. For as a teacher I vowed to make the subject my students and I studied not an end in itself but something that they could then translate into their own lives. Or, as a master teacher once told me, "When you're studying, say, Plato's Republic, *the real subject, the ultimate subject, the only subject that finally matters, is not the treatise of that dead Greek, but that freshman kid in the front row. He or she is your real subject." And in the theatre I vowed never again to direct plays just to entertain the audience, in the limited sense of that word "entertain," but to give them something they could take out of the house, into the street outside the theatre, and weave into the fabric of their own lives. I couldn't say what that would be; each person would have to fashion his or her own postperformance play. And in this way my audience would also become creative. I had gone as the Artist in Residence to the Bone Marrow Unit to give something to the patients. The fact is that they had given me a far greater return on my initial investment.*

CHAPTER 14

Everything Changes

Three years later the head of the Arts in Medicine Program asked me if I would object to being transferred from the Bone Marrow Unit to the Youth Psychiatric Ward on the hospital's eighth floor. Here were housed young people whose problems were so profound that they could no longer live at home but, instead, required round-the-clock treatment at the hospital. Their length of stay ranged from a week to years. This would be a challenge, that was clear, but also a chance to adopt a whole new family.

"We heard you're going to a new place on floor eight," was Freddie's greeting when I arrived on Friday.

"Yes, I am."

No response; the silence was maddening.

"But the person taking my place is fantastic."

"Yeah, I bet he's better than you," an anonymous voice called out from the crowd. It was followed by sarcastic variations of my weak attempt to assure them with "fantastic."

"Everything changes . . . I'm gonna miss you," and then I added a bold "too." More silence. I needed to improvise quickly. "I remember how I felt when I had to leave home for college. I mean, my college was only a few hours' drive away, but it might just as well have been a million miles for all I knew. I didn't want to leave my home. To tell you the truth, I didn't want to leave my father—and my mother." More silence. "Look at it this way. I'm going to the eighth floor, and soon you'll be leaving the hospital."

"We wish!"

My window of opportunity came when Grant asked, "You left home to go to college? My brother stayed right here in Gainesville so he could go to the university. Why didn't you do the same?"

"Well, to tell you the truth. I didn't want to leave home. I didn't even want to go to college. I wanted to become a telephone installer like my dad, and work with him as his assistant. But I left home because my mother made me."

"Made you?"

"Have I ever told you the story called **After Scotty***?"*

"You know you haven't."

No one in my neighborhood went to college. No one in my family had ever gone to college. When I graduated from high school, I looked forward, after a summer job, to starting in the fall as an apprentice installer with my father as teacher in the

Bell Telephone Company. Halfway during the two-week break between the end of the summer job and my new job with the phone company Mother "struck."

In my family we all rose early, for Mother said that, "getting up at five builds character." During the break, however, I had been allowed to sleep late, on the assumption that my character would not seriously degenerate within the short space of two weeks. Yet the third morning Mother came charging into my bedroom at five with her usual "Rise and shine!" She parted the curtains and flung open the windows, all this accompanied by the repetitive "Rise and shine, Sidney!" Now there was what we would call in the theatre a subtext to that "rise and shine," a meaning below the actual words. Something like, "Get out of bed, go out into the world, don't waste a minute, make something of yourself. Be something more than your dad, something better than 'just a telephone worker'!" As "rise and shine" penetrated my consciousness, I cursed her under my pillow, angry that my sole vacation from the family routine was being violated.

"Aw, Mom, why do I have to get up?"

"You're going to Princeton, that's why."

"What's Princeton?"

The night before, on her way home from a friend's house, Mother had stopped by Leary's Book Store—she was into those self-help, Norman Vincent Peale books just becoming popular in the 1950s. It just so happened that Leary's was having a special sale on novels by F. Scott Fitzgerald. Probably because she couldn't resist a bargain, my mother had bought a copy of his

Far Side of Paradise, set at Princeton, where Fitzgerald went as an undergraduate. Apparently, Mother stayed up all night reading and, impressed with Fitzgerald's account of a university whose graduates went on to success in the world as lawyers, doctors, politicians, and major American authors, in fact, whose own president, Woodrow Wilson, had become President of the United States, sure that her own son's going to Princeton would be his salvation from becoming "only a telephone worker," she had made up her mind that, this morning, we would travel to Princeton, New Jersey. By her own fiat she would make me part of that glorious world. With no family history of college and therefore being unfamiliar with the application process, Mother fancied that on the strength of her own personality, carried there by nothing beyond her own will, I would go, like Scott Fitzgerald, to Princeton. I would follow in his footsteps.

"Rise and shine, Sidney. We're leaving in thirty minutes." And in thirty minutes there we were, on August 15, 1956, mother driving the 1938 Dodge. Beside her, with DA-haircut, pimples, and, in the style of the period, peg-pants and a pink jacket, I sat, a nervous, six-foot-one boy, looking ever so much like his dad, next to a four-foot-ten slender woman, with bright red hair, an intense face, and a mind already celebrating her son's success.

In two hours we pulled up to Nassau Hall, Princeton's administration building, once the headquarters of George Washington during the Battle of Trenton and still bearing cannonball scars on its walls. With me literally in tow, one determined woman and one scared kid made their way past boys in tweedy coats and button-down collars, smoking pipes. Mother marched me into the first office she could find, that of Walter Harrison, Dean of Admissions, paying no attention to his secretaries who called out fruitless orders to stop. She charged right into the Dean's inner office.

Before us sat the quintessential Ivy Leaguer—pipe, dark blue jacket with gold sleeve buttons and discrete suede elbow patches. Standing in front of a huge bookcase, Dean Harrison waved away two hovering secretaries and in a serene, measured voice introduced himself as Walter Harrison, no need among those confident aristocrats of the Big 3, as I would realize later, for a title like Dean or Professor or Doctor. In a beautifully cultivated voice he asked, "Madam, what may I do for you?"

In her unmistakable Philly accent, one similar to the Brooklyn accent but with a cacophony of its own special inflections, my mother announced theatrically, "Pleased to meet you, Mr. Harrison. I'm May Elaine Homan; this is my son Sidney. He's bright and he's got talent. I know you're gonna like him!" She was an Auntie Mame, the quintessential stage mother; for her, he was a producer looking over the talent, and I, the boy performer, who, be assured, could act, sing, dance—*and roller-skate!* Mother was reverting to her earlier career as an actress, a shadowy life of run-down theatres and grubby agents that she had known before meeting my father. Confronted with an unfamiliar situation, a totally new character in this Dean of Admissions, she had recast the strange as the familiar.

"Mrs. Homan, why don't you have a seat in the outer office, and I'll be glad to talk with your boy"—"boy" as in "boys," the current word for undergraduates in those days. My mother was flustered. Clearly, she wanted to remain with me as my agent during the interview, but how could she resist such a charming man, one with manners, with bearing, with a style of speaking that seemed both foreign and wondrous? Reluctantly, almost petulantly, she rose with an "all right, if you insist" embossed in every slow movement. A dramatic cross to the door, a reluctant hand on the knob, and then the inevitable exit line. "I'll tell you this, Harrison, you'll like the kid. He's got talent."

The moment I was sure she was gone, I learned forward in my chair. "Dean Harrison, I'm sorry my mother was so . . . well . . . forward."

That kindly man, who would later become a dear friend, replied, "On the contrary, Mr. Homan, I find your mother quite refreshing. You see, I spend most of my day speaking to stuffy matrons from Scarsdale."

While Mother waited anxiously outside, I spent the next hour being interviewed by this genteel figure, a success, to judge by the book-lined office, the gold-leaf paperweight on the desk, the dedicatory plaques on the walls; a success for certain, witnessed by his style, by the grace with which he made me feel comfortable. "Let's talk about matters, shall we, Mr. Homan? I want to find out your opinion on things." Something happened that never happened to kids in my neighborhood: An adult had asked me my opinion, had engaged me in serious conversation, had treated me as an equal. Prose, elegant prose, passionate prose that I had never heard before poured from my lips as I told him about my life, my hopes, about my father the telephone installer, as I joked, for the first time I can remember, about my mother, telling him of *Far Side of Paradise* and my rude awakening earlier that morning, about playing stickball with my cousin Grace who was six feet tall and looked like a boy, about Leslie Doober, Bruzzy Fleck, Connie, Arson, and Fingers Grittle.

Walking to the door—I feared that my mother would have her ear glued to the other side—he turned to me with, "I want you to fill out this application and have your high school send me your transcript as soon as you can. OK? You'll be hearing from me."

In four weeks I received a letter of acceptance from Princeton. As I would learn later, mine was a "special admission." In those days Princeton's undergraduates were overwhelmingly alumni sons, white, Anglo-Saxon, Protestant boys of wealthy families. There were no women, only a few blacks and Latinos, no recognizable minorities to speak of. I was admitted, therefore, as the "token" tough white kid from the inner city. In the next few years, of course, the civil rights movement and then the Vietnam protests would change Princeton, change what Scott Fitzgerald himself once called "the great country club in the sky."

Years later, when I became a Professor of English, once each month my father would call me, and our conversation at some point would invariably lead to the following interchange:

"Sid, you went to Princeton, right?"

"Yes, Dad."

"And the other boys in your class, they all became lawyers and doctors, right?" Now the idea here was that they had gone on to really important professions, to "manly" work, whereas a teacher, let alone a Professor of English, was somehow less significant, perhaps even "unmanly."

"That's right, Dad," I would reply, not wanting to argue.

But Dad would persist. "You know, Sid, having gone to a fine school like Princeton, you could still change your profession, become one of those doctors or lawyers, couldn't you?"

"I could, Dad," was my noncommittal response, sometimes sweetened, as he grew older and sadder, by a "I'm thinking about that."

But after a digression to other topics, Dad would return to my having gone to Princeton, his voice now more mellow.

"You know, Sid, I look at it this way. You're a Professor of English and I'm a telephone installer, right?"

"Right."

"Well, boy, we're both in communications, right?"

"Right, dad."

CHAPTER 15

Last Day on Charlie's Corner

For my last Wednesday on Charlie's Corner, I decided to tell a story that would be something like that final display of fireworks on July 4, when, instead of individual shots, twenty or more fireworks are launched simultaneously, a grand finale that announces both the end and a review of everything seen so far. I would tell a story that had a collage of motifs, like that vegetable soup my mother always kept boiling on the back right burner of our stove. There, in an enormous kettle, would be whatever we had not finished from the last meal, as well as any item in the refrigerator that she thought was coming to the end of its useful life. To supplement my father's income, my mom had worked as a waitress at the Casa Argenio Restaurant, and had observed that its vegetable soup, prized among the patrons who came from all over Philly, was in point of fact a composite of good stock items but, no less, scrapings from customers' plates, all this justified by the head chef with the argument that the constant boiling removed all germs. So I would offer a literary vegetable soup. My own final display, my way of leaving to the kids all the issues that, in retrospect, I saw in my own life, growing up in Philly, till the very moment when I left home. I would tell them the story of **The Casa Argenio**.

⟿⟀⟿

Casa Argenio, House of the Argenio, the enormous restaurant owned and run by the Argenio family—old Ernesto, his wife Delia, and their eight children—had a main dining room that could seat 200 and two banquet rooms holding even more. In the intimate "Virginia Room," named after the sole Argenio daughter, eight lucky diners could gather around a teakwood table, while in the "Grand Ballroom" it was reported a record 400 Elks once grazed. My mother worked as a waitress to supplement my father's income. Since she believed that work built character, at age fifteen I went to work as a pantry boy—for the grand sum of one dollar an hour.

Behind the scenes, behind those swinging doors through which no customer ever passed, stretched the labyrinth of kitchens, "hot" and "cold" pantries, cleaning rooms (three rooms, connected by large archways, where dishes, glasses, and silverware journeyed on conveyor belts through cave-like washing machines), storerooms, and offices. With the exception of "old Mitchell" who did the glasses and "Chef," a large, easily angered, red-haired Swede, the workers behind those doors, the other chefs, the washers, and the janitors, were all African-Americans. Out front, the waitresses, all white, were a motley group, from

"Wild Penny" with enormous bosoms, to mean-spirited "Tex" barely four feet tall, to grandmotherly Emma—young and old, most of them divorced, waitresses who in their pursuit of tips could be as charming to the customers as they were sharp-tongued and competitive behind those swinging doors.

Every day was busy at the Casa Argenio. Starting at 6 AM, the breakfast customers would later meld imperceptibly with those coming for lunches. Dinner extended from five until the last customer left. On the weekends crowds doubled. In the banquet rooms were the Kiwanis on Tuesdays, Rotary Club on Wednesdays, Chamber of Commerce on Thursdays, and Elks on Fridays. Weekends were for wedding receptions and anniversary parties, bridal showers, and, in season, high school graduations.

Presiding over all this was the old man, Ernesto Argenio, a Mafia-like figure now slightly senile, driven to work in a gaudy cream-colored Cadillac by Delia, his plump wife of fifty years. In the back seat sat the lovely daughter Virginia, with black hair falling to her waist and enormous green eyes—and I fell in love with her from the start. Ernesto Jr., the oldest son, was the real boss, a sad figure, physically unattractive, a tyrant wanting desperately to be loved. It was his younger brother Freddie everyone loved, the second in command who, glad to have the modest portion of responsibilities doled out by his older brother, proved sympathetic and fair. Freddie ruled his smaller kingdom by kindness, by circumventing Ernesto Jr., and, when all else failed, by bribery. It was Freddie who used to slip me an extra two dollars each night after I told him that I was impressed by the way John L. Lewis ran the coal-miners union and suggested we organize the kitchen staff in a protest for higher wages.

Chef reigned in the kitchen. His beet-red face showed perpetual displeasure. A french fry on the floor, a dirty plate, a bent tablespoon, the slightest disorder in a pantry, an error calling in an order—any one of these drove him mad. Chef cursed, screamed, threw utensils, and pinched necks, but all these, and more, were mere preludes to his ultimate punishment, hurling himself at you, pushing you to the wall with large shoulders that flapped in counterpoint like the wings of an enraged swan. Commit an infraction, and, after such an assault from Chef, you were "shunned" for the day and went unfed.

From the hot kitchen, his kingdom, Chef spied on the dish, glass, and silverware washers in the adjoining rooms. One afternoon, he lumbered towards me, picked up a glass that somehow had escaped unclean, scowled, and plunged my hands into the scalding water. As he held them there, I did my best to suppress a cry of pain. With that beet-red face next to mine, in a low but potent voice he told me the regular glass washer, old Mitchell, poor Mitchell with the twisted spine and bad breath, friendless Mitchell chained to the machine, was all that I could possibly hope to become in life. "And *Mitchell* never leaves a dirty glass!" he screamed as he marched back to the kitchen.

The following day I was "exiled" to the cold pantry, next to the main dining room. There the pantry boy prepared glasses with ice and water, individual butter pats, saucers of coleslaw, pitchers of cream, plates of rolls—the various items that greeted the customers at their table. The scene was out of Chaplin's

Modern Times; No matter how fast I worked I could just barely keep up with the demand. And the waitresses did not like to be kept waiting. They expected those four butter pats or two glasses of water to be there on the counter waiting for them as they swooped through the pantry, tray in hand, eyes on the party of four that had just taken table 3 at station 2. If there were only three butter pats instead of four, if glasses were empty, if you fell behind in any way, they let you know.

The otherwise mellow Emma, the grandmother, had the nasty habit of socking your ear. Lisa specialized in stiff kicks, not one, always two, to the buttocks. Rosa once dragged me into the dining room to apologize to a customer for a partially filled saucer of coleslaw. Two hours in the pantry seemed like eight; dishwashing, even within sight of Chef, a paradise. Two weeks later Freddie took pity on me.

I had just broken a glass in the ice bin and was faced with the enormous task of taking out all the ice, cleaning the bin, checking for broken glass, and refilling the bin, all the while leaving plates crying out for their butter pats and pitchers for their cream. Suddenly Freddie was beside me, the second-in-command now my co-pantry boy. He was a magician, dealing out butter pats as if they were poker chips, arranging a reserve row of water glasses—a luxury of preplanning beyond my abilities.

"Ernesto's just fired the hot-pantry boy. Why don't you take his place, Sid?"

The hot pantry! The promised land. El Dorado! In the hot pantry you had only two responsibilities. One was filling the five large urns, four with coffee, the fifth with hot water for tea.

They were *very* large urns; if you got them into a rotation, or if there wasn't an abnormal demand for coffee, you could count on each urn lasting an hour. It took about five minutes to refill the urn by pouring nine gallons of water through a filter with six pounds of fresh coffee. Your second responsibility was cutting the various pies—apple, blueberry, peach, blackberry, and rhubarb—keeping four plates of each ready for the waitresses. With the coffee brewing and the pies, the place smelled delicious and you didn't have to rush. Also, by the time the waitresses came to the hot pantry their anxiety was gone; they had sized up the customers and knew what their tip would be. From time to time, but only when things were slow, I would emulate my hero Freddie and help out Lynn, the new fellow now imprisoned in the cold pantry.

In the hot pantry I stayed, mastering the trivial details of my new world. On Sundays apple pies outsold the other four varieties two to one. Only senior citizens ordered rhubarb. Peach performed best in summer, and blueberry went faster than blackberry. Buoyed with this knowledge, I became daring, carefree. Within two weeks I had flouted the hot-pantry rule dictating four cut pieces for each variety of pie that Ernesto Jr. once told me was immutable. On the weekends seven apples stood ready at all times, and, except in the summer months, I was able to reduce the available blackberry and even peach to a single piece. Rhubarb, the waitresses soon learned, could be had only on request. The operating principle here was that the less time a pie waited on the counter, the fresher it would be for the customer. What is more, I took pride in not having to throw out coffee at the end of the day. At four on a weekday and at five on the weekend four urns brewed. But on Saturday we would go down to three urns by seven in the evening, two by eight, one by nine. If all went well, that final urn at ten would hold just enough coffee so that the help could get a cup before going home at eleven.

Chef even complimented me on "the state of the pantry," though, picking up a piece of blueberry pie, he groused about its being cut too wide. I could live with that. On television, in one of those fifteen-minute musical segments preceding the evening news, Roberta Quinlan was singing, "Welcome to my world. Won't you come on in?" In imitation, I put a banner over the door with those lyrics. Everyone laughed, even Chef. The dour Ernesto Jr. had it taken down. That same evening, as he slipped me my extra two dollars in pay, Freddie handed me the banner, rolled up, suggesting I display it over my bedroom door. As he walked me out to the parking lot, I saw the gorgeous Virginia Argenio get into a 1955 Chevy Bellaire, white with a red side stripe, driven by a greasy-looking fellow with monstrous sideburns, a toothpick projecting between his teeth. My heart sank.

Early one Saturday morning the kitchen prepared for an onslaught. That evening 300 members of the Philadelphia Gourmet Society were to dine in the Grand Ballroom. Forced to cook according to the group's specifications, given months ago when the Society had made reservations, Chef stormed about the kitchen in an especially foul mood. When I came in at four, he barked at me, "Open the nuts." Before I could get out a "Nuts?" he pointed toward the large, rectangular store-room adjacent to the hot kitchen. "After they're opened, put them in those 300 fancy cups. The cups are on the bottom shelf in the far-right corner. When you've done that, put one cup at each place in the Ballroom. On the right, above the knife!"

Ten very large tins of nuts were waiting for me. No generic brand, the nuts, the label stated proudly, were imported from a "Specialty Grower in Puerto Rico." Obviously these nuts would meet the demanding tastes of the diners who would descend on us that evening. When I opened the first can, however, I almost passed out. It was crawling with little bugs, thousands of them, not so much eating as coexisting with the nuts! A second can. More bugs! A third. Bugs were the rule—that was for sure. I picked up the first can, swarming with the creatures, and took it right to Chef.

His response was blunt. "We've got to serve those nuts. That's what those bastards ordered. There's no time to get new nuts." Then, without hesitation, "You think you're so smart. You figure something out!" With that, Chef stalked behind his serving counter, a place off-limits to anyone but fellow chefs. Freddie, who had overheard all of this from the corner of the kitchen, gave me a fatherly look. "You'll think of something, Sid. There's a dollar bonus in it if you do."

"Make it two, boss?"

"OK, Sid, OK."

Sustained by Freddie's faith and his promise of two extra dol-lars, a half hour later I came up with a plan. I poured the nuts from all ten cans, complete with bugs, onto ten large rectangular trays on which we baked pies. Then I put the trays in the long ovens lining the wall across from the serving counter, and turned up the heat. Chef and his five assistants looked up every once in a while. Grins were exchanged. Fifteen minutes later I opened the oven and took out the trays. The nuts had stayed the same; the bugs, however, had shriveled so much that they now looked like pieces of nuts that had broken off, or maybe flakes of nut skin. Unless you knew my desperate remedy, you would be none the wiser.

That evening, after pointing out to the members of the Gourmet Society that the nuts garnishing the table had been "imported especially from Puerto Rico" for the occasion, the waitresses made much ado in asking the diners how they found the delicacy. Every "tasty" and "delicious" was met with all-knowing winks among the women. Barely able to hold their laughter until they passed through the swinging doors into the kitchen, they would report the compliments verbatim to me and the rest of the staff. Penny was in especially high spirits as she toyed with the gourmet diners.

"Don't you find these nuts have a special taste? You know, something that sets them apart from other gourmet nuts?"

"I wonder how they prepared these nuts. They're so good, and—dumb me!—I always thought once you'd tasted one nut you'd tasted them all."

However, just when I thought I had it made at Casa Argenio, just when I felt secure, my life there changed once more. "You're gonna work with Del," Ernesto Jr. said in his usual laconic fashion when I came to work next Saturday morning. *Del*!

Del was a young black man who came in every Sunday to make coleslaw for the week. No one really knew him. From the moment Del arrived at eight he went down to the third basement for the day, even eating his two meals there, and never came back upstairs until it was time to leave.

Rumors abounded: Del was crazy, he was retarded, he was just a loner. I myself had only seen him from a distance. When he finished a vat of coleslaw, Del would send it up to the main floor by a dumbwaiter. I'd help one of the staff pull out the huge vat, weighing some one hundred pounds, and carry it into the walk-in refrigerator. Thirty minutes later another batch would be ready.

Marvelous coleslaw, creamy, fresh coleslaw, coleslaw so good that people all over the city, if they knew nothing else about Casa Argenio, knew about the coleslaw. Customers, especially our regulars, ordered a pint or quart to take home. While Ernesto Jr. frowned on the "take-out" restaurants just becoming popular in the '50s, he did allow people to come to the back door and place special orders. So far Del alone made coleslaw, but, as Freddie explained, demand had grown so that from now on I would be his helper on Sundays.

That morning I made my way down the steps, past the first basement of dry goods, past the second basement housing linen and cleaning supplies, to the third and final basement. A single light burned in the center of the room; my eyes had trouble adjusting to this nether world. With his back to me, Del stood at the far end of the room. Behind him, to his left, a large vat rested on the table. To his right two bins overflowed with heads of cabbage and lettuce; on the left stood a box of carrots about the size of a coffin. Ahead were shelves with jars of salad dressing, mayonnaise, and boxes of salt and pepper—the ingredients for Casa Argenio's magical coleslaw.

"Hey, Sid, nice to see ya."

Del was in his twenties, slim, lanky, an inch or so shorter than me. In the dim light his skin shown a rich purple, as if he were royalty, and when he went into the cabbage bin for fresh supplies, he melted into the blackness encircling our worktable. Del had enormous eyes, not abnormally so, yet still enormous. His voice, with a thick accent, was soft and assured.

I became his apprentice and he, my patient teacher. The first time I tried to dice a cabbage by placing it squarely on the table and chopping away, Del laughed. "Look, ya hold it in your hand like this, tilt it towards that big bowl there, make five deep slices, almost down to the bottom. See? Don't forget about your hand. Cut thin layers. You got it?"

It took me weeks of Sundays to get to Del's speed, not to mention a few nicks in my hand which I hid from him. Now carrots, there was an art. You held the carrot in one hand, pointing toward the vat and sliced away. When the carrot had been reduced to a stub of about one-half inch, you flung it in the air, slicing it twice as it fell, adding three final pieces to the vat. Perfect carrot slicing took me four lessons.

Nothing mysterious about making coleslaw. You diced two heads of cabbage for every head of lettuce, for a grand total of about eighty pounds, added about thirty carrots, three gallons of mayonnaise, two of salad dressing, and a heavy hand of salt and pepper. Then Del and I would roll up our sleeves and plunge our hands into the mixture to stir it. Finally, we would lift the vat onto the dumbwaiter and sound the signal, and then begin immediately on the next vat.

For two Sundays Del and I worked mostly in silence—all day. We started in the morning, finished in the evening. My beloved Virginia Argenio brought our meals, and would sometimes stay and eat with us. I cherished those times. Del rarely spoke, yet he seemed interested in what we said. Virginia and I talked mainly about the restaurant. The hostess in the main dining room, she shared stories about the customers and the waitresses, while I told about the personalities in the kitchen.

With Virginia I somehow felt at ease. She seemed to enjoy her visits to our quiet place, the air thick with cabbage and mayonnaise. What a strange group we were. Glad to escape the frenzy of the dining room, Virginia would lean back in an old stuffed chair, resting her chin on that slender right hand, long black hair falling over her left shoulder, her voice bright, her expression lively and intense. Del silent, his eyes following the conversation, sometimes would laugh softly, knowing he was accepted, included by both Virginia and me in a conversation in which he never had to join directly. And I, hopelessly in love with Virginia, tried to hide my feelings.

By the third week Del and I were chatting like old buddies. We spoke of coleslaw, and of the people above. As the weeks passed we became more relaxed, more intimate. Del lived in the city, not far, actually, from where I grew up. His was a home without a father, a neighborhood once integrated but now all black, one of street gangs and drugs. Del had a girlfriend who lived with him and his family. She was five months pregnant. In the racially segregated 1950s, before Dr. King or Malcolm X, before the civil rights movement, Del inhabited a world foreign and, for that very reason, exciting to me. I wanted to hear as much about him as he did of me. For him, the more boring my life, the better it seemed to him. That we stayed home Friday nights listening to the radio pleased him. The smallest detail about taking care of our rabbit Thumper or going to the hardware store on Saturday mornings with Dad made him want to hear more.

We hacked and sliced cabbage; we talked and sent carrots flying. We rolled up our sleeves and immersed our hands into the vat, our mission to create for an eager daylight world above that exotic suspension of vegetables and dressings.

I grew to cherish those Sundays with Del. Now, when Virginia came down with our meals, Del was a full partner in our conversations. She supplied us with details of the Argenio family, the latest gossip about her brother's unfaithful wife, news of relatives in the old country, the dark side of old Ernesto's business ventures, petty rivalries, little triumphs of the large Italian family, the latest jokes from the waitresses, even details about Chef that humanized him.

"She has a thing for you," Del observed one day after Virginia had gone upstairs.

"Come on!"

"I know. I got experience with women."

"A thing?"

"Yes."

"What should I do?"

"Just do what ya been doing, man."

"But—"

"You learned how to cut cabbage, didn't you?"

"Yeah."

"Well, you'll be able to handle women. Trust me."

Two young men chatting away, true friends now, pals, white and black hands, black and white arms navigating the creamy sea of coleslaw, sending up vat upon vat; vats begat like the progeny of *Genesis*, vat upon vat journeying from that twilight third world, past the linen and cleaning supplies of the second basement, past the foodstuffs, the gallons of canned peaches and apples of the first basement, delivered from the expectant dumbwaiter into waiting arms. Casa Argenio coleslaw, made from the loving hands of Del and Sid, famous throughout the city, recommended by none other than the Mayor of Philadelphia himself, endorsed by the Governor, making its way to diners about to devour breaded-veal cutlets smothered in Ernesto Argenio's own "original spaghetti sauce." Moms and pops wiped plump Delia's apple pie from their lips, then carried home the coleslaw with the reverence priests accord the chalice, the coleslaw gracing the next day's meal, and the one after, and the one after, until the next pilgrimage to the House of Argenio. Casa Argenio coleslaw, made by Del and Sid, bought, sold, cherished, carried home; take-outs from the son of a Mafia-boss who scorned take-outs; the cabbage, lettuce, carrots, mayonnaise, salad dressing, and salt and pepper in perfect suspension;

coleslaw spreading beyond Casa Argenio, beyond the city, beyond Pennsylvania, beyond the tranquil America of the Eisenhower years; coleslaw for the World!

"You'll be able to handle women. Trust me." The kindly prediction from this man about to become a father himself stayed with me all day, and his were the last words I thought of as I fell asleep late at night, exhausted from thirteen hours of making coleslaw, my hands, despite five washings, still fragrant with cabbage and salad dressing.

Each year the Argenios staged a party for the employees at their palatial home. On their well-manicured lawn stood tables bursting with food. A huge bowl of our coleslaw served as a centerpiece. Unshackled from those starched-white uniforms with the Argenio crest of arms emblazoned above their left breasts, the waitresses looked resplendent, although Penny's tacky, low-cut dress brought stares and more than a few snide comments. Tex brought a lasso and regaled us with tricks from her girlhood. Wine flowed freely. Even Ernesto Jr. managed an expression approaching a grimace. Chef, his usual solemn self, put on a pained smile when someone reminded him about the incident with the bug-infested nuts.

As the day went on, class distinctions broke down. Lynn, the new pantry boy, played ping-pong with ancient Delia as his partner. Freddie showed old Mitchell the Italian game of bocce. The restaurant stood abandoned. On this festive day no butter pats would wait in formation for the waitresses on their way to that table of four in the Main Room. Today no Elk would dip his freshly baked roll in creamed chicken. Not today. Today, that single bulb in the third basement was off. Today, we let down our collective hair.

Late in the afternoon the games began. In silly ones like "the Wheelbarrow" you held up someone by the legs while their hands served as wheels, or in "the Egg" people maneuvered on their hands and knees as they pushed an egg along the ground to the finish line. Freddie announced the "Three-Leg Race," where contestants, arms around each other, their three left legs tied together in front of them, tried to make it across the finish line.

I had seen Virginia, shared a drink with her for a few minutes, and another time joined her conversation. Despite's Del's comment, I feared making a fool of myself. Now she came up to Del and me with, "Come on, coleslaw partners, let's make a team for the three-leg race!"

Under Freddie's instructions, we bunched together, with Virginia between Del and me, propping our left legs on a chair while Tex tied them together. "Get ready," Freddie warned as awkwardly, comically, we joined the other contestants at the starting line, the combined left legs dangling before us like the antennae of a praying mantis. We fell twice, and needed help balancing ourselves, all this, of course, to howls of laughter.

"Let's get closer together so we won't wobble so much," Virginia suggested as we took our positions. I could feel her face now pressed against mine, my right arm around her shoulder, and Del's arms embracing the both of us. The gun sounded. We were off!

Of the five entries, we soon fell to last place, but we didn't care. We lost the race; we never made it to the finish line. We lay there, three as one, black and white arms and legs helplessly, absurdly, wonderfully intertwined. As we got up, I felt Virginia's hand brush against my cheek before she disappeared into the crowd. Del smiled at me.

Delia Argenio came up. After a few pleasantries, she asked Del where his girlfriend was.

"She wasn't feeling so well, Mrs. Argenio. You know, the baby might come any day now so my mom's looking after her. But she'll be fine."

With that, the band started playing, and Mrs. Argenio—*Mrs. Argenio*, of all people!—asked me to dance. I blushed, but what could I do? I caught a strange smile from Del. Minutes later Virginia started dancing with him, and, in the 1950s, you must remember what a bold move that was. Would I get a chance to dance with her? Should I ask her?

Fortunately, I didn't have to make that decision. The waitresses had decided to turn the tables on the men, and so the women took the lead in picking dance partners. I had all sorts of partners, from Penny, who couldn't have been more than twenty-two, to Emma, the grandmother. Spurred on by Virginia's example earlier, black chefs and kitchen staff danced with white waitresses. Selma, "I have a dream," Reverend Jesse Jackson, the campus protests—these were years away. Flushed with wine, we danced, all of us. Slow dance, jitterbug, shaking our hips to Elvis, doing the twist with Little Richard, Mafia Ernesto leading us in a wine-stomping dance from the old country. Skirts ballooned. Clutching an apron from the kitchen, Penny did a parody of the fan dance. Lynn, liberated this day from the cold pantry, imitated Fabian. Partners held each other tightly, only to be parted by someone breaking in. Even Chef tapped his foot. Prodded by Delia, Ernesto Jr. danced with his own wife. That was a first! The tables were replenished by scouts sent to plunder the restaurant's walk-in freezer. Anthony, the youngest Argenio, demonstrated how to pour a gallon jug of wine while holding it over your shoulder. Jokes rippled through the crowd. Tongues slurred greetings. Makeup ran, and men unbuttoned their shirts. When it became dark, Freddie lit luminaries around the lawn. Virginia stood alone, listening to the band.

I got up my nerve. "Virginia, would you like to dance?'

"I've been waiting all evening for you to ask me."

We had a word in the 1950s for what I felt, "thrill," the staple of countless popular songs.

As I tried to make up an excuse for not asking her earlier, she silenced me with a simple "Come on, you dope. You don't need to explain."

Virginia was my only partner for the rest of the evening. We held each other tightly, saying little.

"One more dance," Ernesto Jr. announced at midnight.

My lips pressed against Virginia; I could smell her hair.

At the end of the night we clung to each other until the lights went on. Mrs. Argenio whisked Virginia away. I stood for a while in the center of the yard, transfixed. Del came up.

"I was right, man."

"Yeah, you were right," I said sheepishly as we exchanged knowing smiles.

"See you next Sunday."

"No, remember—I'm going away to college."

"Oh, yeah, I forgot." I saw a sadness in Del's eyes. Then he recovered. "Listen, man, you'll be a winner there too. Just don't forget me."

"Forget you? Hell, you taught me how to cut cabbage! Forget you?" We laughed and then embraced, embraced in a time long before it was deemed acceptable for men. I couldn't hold back my tears.

"Come on!" Freddie called out from the parking lot.

Two days later, just an hour before my parents and I left for Princeton, Freddie called to say good-bye. He also had bad news. Del's baby had died at birth. Freddie didn't know the cause, only that the baby had died.

That evening, after all the excitement of moving into my dorm had died down, I wrote to Del, telling him how sad I felt about the baby, reminding him of my promise not to forget him, and saying that, whatever happened to me in life, nothing would be as special as our working together down in that third basement making coleslaw. I didn't know his address, so I sent the letter care of Freddie at Casa Argenio. I knew that good man would make sure it got to Del.

⁓⚜⁓

When I finished the head nurse appeared, a bit annoyed at me that the long story would now make her patients late for dinner. Despite her commands that the kids get back to their rooms, they swarmed around me, with hugs and kisses. They said very little. Hugs and kisses substituted for words, were "more than words can witness," as Shakespeare once said. The trip back up the hill to my car was harder than ever before.

Next Friday I would go to the Youth Psychiatric Ward where there would be a different audience. I looked forward to meeting them.

Six months after starting on the new ward, I paid a visit to my friend John Graham-Pole.

"I hear you're doing well with the teenagers on the eighth floor."

I handed John a manuscript copy of the stories from the Bone Marrow Unit. "For you, John, my friend."

"I'll tell you what, Sid, I'll make a Xerox copy, and we'll put it in a binder on the table in Charlie's Corner. Beats those out-of-date magazines you find in doctors' offices, right?"

"Right."

A year later I dropped by Charlie's Corner. It was deserted. The same rug. The same clock. The same unfinished puzzle. But there, on the table, I saw that the binder of my stories was open. Someone had been reading **A Fish in the Moonlight**. I smiled—and was grateful.